W9-AZL-773

Occupational Medicine

Risk and Disability Evaluation in the Workplace

Guest Editors:

David C. Randolph, MD, MPH, FAADEP
Fellow, American Academy of Disability Evaluating Physicians
Fellow, American College of Occupational Medicine
Consultant, Occupational Medicine and Disability Determination
Milford, Ohio

Mohammed I. Ranavaya, MD, MS, FAADEP, CIME
Professor, Division of Occupational and Environmental Medicine
Chief, Division of Disability Medicine
Department of Family and Community Health
Marshall University School of Medicine
Huntington, West Virginia

Volume 15/Number 4
HANLEY & BELFUS, INC.

October–December 2000
Philadelphia

STATE OF THE ART REVIEWS

Publisher: HANLEY & BELFUS, INC.
Medical Publishers
210 South 13th Street
Philadelphia, PA 19107
(215) 546-4995
Fax (215) 790-9330
Web site: http:/www.hanleyandbelfus.com

OCCUPATIONAL MEDICINE: State of the Art Reviews is indexed in *Index Medicus/MEDLINE, BioSciences Information Service, Current Contents* and *ISI/BIOMED, CINAHL database, and Cumulative Index to Nursing & Allied Health Literature.* Printed on acid-free paper.

Authorization to photocopy items for internal or personal use, or the internal or personal use of specific clients, is granted by Hanley & Belfus, Inc. for libraries and other users registered with the Copyright Clearance Center (CCC) Transaction Reporting Service, provided that the base fee of $1.00 per copy plus $0.25 per page is paid directly to the CCC, 222 Rosewood Drive, Danvers, MA 01923. Identify this publication by including with your payment the fee code, 0885-114X/00 $1.00 + .25.

OCCUPATIONAL MEDICINE: State of the Art Reviews   ISSN 0885-114X
October–December 2000   Volume 15, Number 4   ISBN 1-56053-328-5

OCCUPATIONAL MEDICINE: State of the Art Reviews is published quarterly by Hanley & Belfus, Inc., 210 South 13th Street, Philadelphia, Pennsylvania 19107. Periodical postage paid at Philadelphia, PA, and at additional mailing offices.

POSTMASTER: Send address changes to OCCUPATIONAL MEDICINE: State of the Art Reviews, Hanley & Belfus, Inc., 210 South 13th Street, Philadelphia, PA 19107.

The 2000 subscription price is $96.00 per year U.S., $106.00 outside U.S. (add $40.00 for air mail).

Occupational Medicine: State of the Art Reviews
Vol. 15, No. 4, October–December 2000

RISK AND DISABILITY EVALUATION IN THE WORKPLACE
Edited by David C. Randolph, MD, MPH, FAADEP, and
Mohammed I. Ranavaya, MD, MS, FAADEP, CIME

CONTENTS

The significance of neuromusculoskeletal conditions in the workplace is the subject of much discussion among occupational medicine professionals. There are differing philosophies as to what constitutes appropriate diagnostic criteria for identification of these conditions. The traditional diagnostic model requires the presence of objective pathology. An emerging symptom-based model accepts that symptoms by themselves can constitute a diagnostic entity. The extent to which these conditions are considered to be associated with occupational activity depends greatly upon which of the two models is employed. This chapter presents an overview of each diagnostic model and a discussion of the impact each has on the prevalence of identified conditions and the manner in which the various diagnostic requirements can affect treatment, prevention, and disability rating protocols. **Occup Med 15:677–693, 2000.**

A review of national statistics and recent studies strongly suggests that current administrative and medical systems, when applied to managing workers' compensation claims and other disability-related benefit programs, are often ineffective and costly, and can even promote disability. With numerous medical and occupational health articles published daily, it is difficult to develop practical strategies for daily management of disability claims that make use of current information. It is the authors' view that a comprehensive, dynamic model for management exists within the military's "Forward Treatment" methodology. This model, originally published in *The Journal of Occupational Rehabilitation,* has been expanded to include those methods demonstrated in literature to both reduce claims and deal with them in an efficient, fair, and timely manner. Because military personnel and employed individuals are similarly entitled, the military's proven model can be effective in reducing claim rates and costs associated with workers' compensation as well as short- and long-term disability programs. The model, given the acronym S.P.I.C.E., includes five components: Simplicity, Proximity, Immediacy, Centrality, and Expectancy. **Occup Med 15:695–722, 2000.**

Fitness statements often are required of physicians by patients, employers, governmental agencies, and insurance providers to determine if the patient is fit for duty. Physicians making these ability statements are legally obligated to carefully justify them when placing or excluding individuals from the workplace. The Americans with Disabilities Act (ADA) mandates that medical providers use justifiable criteria and rational thought when determining the capability and risk of an individual. This chapter reviews the legal requirements of the ADA for employers and physicians and presents a uniform methodology that both can use to determine the performance capability of an individual with a temporary or permanent impairment or disability. **Occup Med 15:723–737, 2000.**

Abnormal illness behaviors, ranging from non-deliberate distortion to intentional deception, are associated with clinical phenomena that lie along a continuum from unconscious symptom exaggeration to psychiatric disorders and malingering. Failure to recognize abnormal illness behavior leads to inappropriate treatment and erroneous estimates of impairment or disability. This review is divided into three sections. First, basic terms are defined, including dissimulation, distortion, deception, misattribution, false imputation, and malingering. Second, syndromes characterized by abnormal illness behavior are described, including somatization, somatoform disorders, factitious disorders, and symptom magnification. Third, methods for detecting deception are illustrated, including maximum voluntary effort assessment, objective personality inventories, and symptom validity testing. **Occup Med 15:739–754, 2000.**

Chronic pain has become a major public health problem. Often, the availability of entitlement programs as well as psychosocial, occupational, and other nonmedical factors—rather than objective pathophysiology—are major contributors to disability. In this chapter, the authors discuss the relationship between impairment and disability and detail factors likely to predict or contribute to adverse clinical outcome and disability. Guidelines for disability prevention also are examined. **Occup Med 15:755–770, 2000.**

The assessment and management of occupational and nonoccupational injuries and illnesses of the extremities require knowledge of the same concepts of impairment and disability that are used when evaluating or treating problems of other body systems. Dr. Talmage discusses the need for an accurate and objectively verifiable diagnosis and focuses on upper extremity pain in workers and the term "tendinitis." The concept of maximal medical improvement is considered, with examples of knee injuries to the menisci and localized articular cartilage defects. Causation controversies are explored using carpal tunnel syndrome as the example. The impairment rating process is illustrated by use of the *AMA Guides* system. A "checklist" to insure completeness of the examination of extremity problems is offered. Disability assessment and management is discussed, with an emphasis on the difference between abilities (capacities) and risk-based restrictions. The author concludes with thoughts on how to minimize disability. **Occup Med 15:771–788, 2000.**

Worksite Disability Management Model for Effective Return-to-Work Planning

Donald E. Shrey

The growth of disability management programs represents a paradigm shift from traditional clinic-based rehabilitation services to worksite-based interventions that dramatically reduce lost time and costs. Supportive policies and steps in the return-to-work process are illustrated, from the point of worker injury and early intervention, through work ability assessment, return-to-work planning, job-site accommodation, and successful return to work. Creative return-to-work options, including "job banks," are discussed as practical methods to facilitate the worker's gradual return to full duty status while completing the medical recovery process. Worker, worksite, and community resource factors related to return-to-work outcomes are discussed. **Occup Med 15:789–801, 2000.**

Timothy Proctor, Robert J. Gatchel, Richard C. Robinson

This article reviews the research on the risk of pain and disability due to psychosocial variables. Variables such as general distress, psychopathology, depression, abuse, and catastrophizing are discussed in relation to the risk of disability. Ways to conceptualize the complex relationships among pain, disability, and several psychosocial variables are also explored. In addition, the identification of adaptive and of protective ways to manage pain and decrease the risk of disability is highlighted. Finally, the authors recommend areas for future research. **Occup Med 15: 803–812, 2000.**

David C. Randolph

Functional testing has evolved to a new sophistication, and is currently used in a variety of situations to assist the employer and physician in safely placing an individual at the job site. The functional capacity evaluation can be employed in several ways, not only to place individuals safely in jobs, but also to monitor their progress throughout recovery from an injury or illness and aid in the establishment of vocational counseling and planning. Many legal issues now alter employer techniques for hiring and assigning people to jobs. This state of affairs places increasing importance on functional testing. **Occup Med 15:813–821, 2000.**

CONTRIBUTOR LIST

Gerald M. Aronoff, MD
Assistant Clinical Professor, Department of Psychiatry, Tufts Medical School, Boston, Massachusetts

Thomas Scott Campion, PT
Director of Physical Therapy, Presbyterian Rehabilitation Services, Charlotte, North Carolina

Alan Lawrence Colledge, MD
Medical Director, Labor Commission of Utah, Salt Lake City, Utah

Leon H. Ensalada, MD, MPH
President, Leon Ensalada & Associates, Hendersonville, Tennessee

Jeffrey B. Feldman, PhD
Assistant Professor, Section of Neuropsychology, Department of Neurology, Wake Forest University School of Medicine, Winston-Salem, North Carolina

Robert J. Gatchel, PhD
Professor, Department of Psychiatry, University of Texas Southwestern Medical Center, Dallas, Texas

Richard E. Johns, Jr., MD, MSPH
Alliant Techsystems, Magna, Utah

Hugh I. Johnson, MPA
Risk Manager, Utah Transit Authority, Salt Lake City, Utah

Kenneth D. Meadows, PT
Chief Physical Therapist, Portland Hand Surgery and Rehabilitation Center, Portland, Oregon

Peter A. Nathan, MD
Portland Hand Surgery and Rehabilitation Center, Portland, Oregon

Timothy Proctor
PhD Candidate, Department of Psychiatry, University of Texas Southwestern Medical Center, Dallas, Texas

David C. Randolph, MD, MPH, FAADEP
Fellow, American Academy of Disability Evaluating Physicians; Fellow, American College of Occupational Medicine; Consultant, Occupational Medicine and Disability Determination, Milford, Ohio

Richard C. Robinson, PhD
Postdoctoral Fellow, Department of Psychiatry, University of Texas Southwestern Medical Center, Dallas, Texas

Donald E. Shrey, PhD, CRC
Associate Professor, Department of Physical Medicine and Rehabilitation, University of Cincinnati Medical Center, Cincinnati, Ohio

James B. Talmage, MD
Medical Director, Occupational Health Center, Cookeville Regional Medical Center, Cookeville, Tennessee.

PUBLISHED ISSUES
(*available from the publisher*)

2001 ISSUES

Municipal Workers
Edited by Peter Orris, MD
Cook County Hospital
Chicago, Illinois
and Karen Mulloy, DO
University of New Mexico
Albuquerque, New Mexico

Nuclear Energy Industry
Edited by Gregg Wilkinson, PhD
State University of New York
Buffalo, New York

The Management Perspective
Edited by L. Fleming Fallon, Jr., MD
Bowling Green State University
Bowling Green, Ohio

Health Hazards in the Arts
Edited by Katherine Duvall, MD and
  David Hinkamp, MD
The Arts-Medicine Project
University of Illinois
Chicago, Illinois

2000 ISSUES

**The Workplace and Cardiovascular
Disease**
Edited by Peter Schnall, MD, MPH
and Dean Baker, MD, MPH
University of California, Irvine, California;
Paul Landsbergis, PhD, EdD, MPH
Cornell University, New York, New York;
Karen Belkić, MD, PhD
University of Southern California
Los Angeles, California

Occupational Asthma
Edited by Daniel E. Banks, MD
and Mei-Lin Wang, MD
West Virginia University
Morgantown, West Virginia

**Multiple Chemical Sensitivity/
Idiopathic Environmental Intolerance**
Edited by Patricia J. Sparks, MD, MPH
Private Consultant
Occupational and Environmental
  Medicine
Mercer Island, Washington

**Risk and Disability Evaluation
in the Workplace**
Edited by David C. Randolph, MD, MPH
Occupational Medicine Physician
  and Consultant
Private Practice
Cincinnati, Ohio
and Mohammed I. Ranavaya, MD, MS
Marshall University
Huntington, West Virginia

1999 ISSUES

Office Ergonomics
Edited by Martin Cherniack, MD, MPH
University of Connecticut
Farmington, Connecticut

Animal Handlers
Edited by Ricky L. Langley, MD, MPH
North Carolina Department of Health
  and Human Services
Raleigh, North Carolina

Special Populations
Edited by Howard Frumkin, MD
Emory University, Atlanta, Georgia
and Glenn Pransky, MD, MOccH
University of Massachusetts
Worcester, Massachusetts

**Health Issues in the Plastics
and Rubber Industries**
Edited by Richard Lewis, MD, MPH
University of Louisville,
Louisville, Kentucky

Ordering Information:
Subscriptions for full year and single issues are available from the publishers—
Hanley & Belfus, Inc., 210 South 13th Street, Philadelphia, PA 19107
Telephone (215) 546-7293; (800) 962-1892. Fax (215) 790-9330. Website www.hanleyandbelfus.com

PREFACE

All medical professionals involved in occupational health issues are aware of the burgeoning problems centered on disability. These issues range from the mundane (filling out forms, coding diagnoses, and estimating return-to-work dates) to the professionally challenging tasks of dealing with chronically disabling conditions. Clearly, some conditions lend themselves to the development of long-term disability more than others. Some of the former have been identified and presented in this text to allow the reader to become more familiar with the "state of the art" thinking with respect to these diagnoses. Various disabling extremity conditions are reviewed by Talmage; cumulative trauma disorders of the upper extremities are examined by Nathan and Meadows; and chronic pain is addressed by Aronoff and Campion.

There are times, especially in today's society, when management of disability is problematic due to claims administration rather than provision of care. Colledge and Johns discuss a novel approach to state workers' compensation systems. Colledge is a principle author and administrator of the Utah workers' compensation system; he has been instrumental in reconstructing that system and administering it into a highly successful, well-recognized, and respected mechanism for the management of work-related health problems. Physicians and other healthcare workers who may be embroiled in disability systems mired in bureaucracy may gain substantial insight in the article by Colledge and Johnson. The "SPICE" system has a proven and recognized track record from which we may all gain practical pointers to improve the functioning of our own systems.

We have all had occasions to evaluate and treat individuals whose physical presentation is inconsistent with the pathologic features for which they are being treated. Ensalada provides an excellent guide to the evaluation of "illness behavior," with a summary of the tools available to practitioners to evaluate the physical and emotional factors associated with such presentations. Along these lines, I provide a discussion on the current state of the art of functional testing, and explore its usefulness from a practical standpoint to evaluate individuals involved in the treatment and rehabilitative phase of their clinical problems. Functional testing is becoming more and more controversial. This article describes the current tools available, as well as the theoretical aspects of these tools. This information, especially when combined with that provided by Colledge and Johns in their "unified fitness report" article, addresses multiple concerns regarding worker abilities.

Proctor, Gatchell, and Robinson provide an overview of psychosocial risk factors that can lead to the development of disabling conditions. Their presentation of these issues, combined with their clear clinical and practical perspective, allow a good, comprehensive evaluation not only of these crucial mental health problems, but also the risk evolving from such problems.

Shrey addresses employment and vocational risk from the employer's perspective. This represents a somewhat different view, but enables healthcare providers to evaluate these issues from a different stance and provides better insight into the process of vocational rehabilitation.

Long-term, disabling health problems pose a problem for healthcare providers in a variety of different fashions. The risk of developing long-term disability substantially escalates if the players in this process (healthcare providers, employer representatives, legal representatives, as well as the injured or ill worker) are unaware of all aspects of the pathophysiology and nuances of the treatments available.

Individual healthcare professionals, be they physicians, case managers, or human resource personnel or administrators, are better equipped to handle the risk of long-term disability when they are familiar with the issues surrounding disability conditions. This compendium is directed toward that educational process. It is hoped that the information contained in these articles will provide the reader with greater insight into contemporary issues and assist in evaluating risks and, when possible, avoiding long-term disability.

David C. Randolph, MD, MPH, FAADEP
Mohammed I. Ranavaya, MD, MS, FAADEP, CIME
EDITORS

PETER A. NATHAN, MD
KENNETH D. MEADOWS, PT

NEUROMUSCULOSKELETAL CONDITIONS OF THE UPPER EXTREMITY: ARE THEY DUE TO REPETITIVE OCCUPATIONAL TRAUMA?

From Portland Hand Surgery and
   Rehabilitation Center
   Portland, Oregon

Reprint requests to:
   Peter A. Nathan, MD
   Portland Hand Surgery and
   Rehabilitation Center
   2455 N.W. Marshall, Suite 1
   Portland, OR 97210-2997

Repetitive use of the hands is part of the everyday experience. Symptoms of the upper extremity are common and can develop during work or recreation, and even in the absence of vigorous physical activity. These symptoms often are transient and may not represent tissue pathology. Persistent symptoms can alert us to an underlying pathologic condition. Diagnosis and treatment may be pursued when the symptomatic experience is interpreted as reflecting an underlying medical condition. Verbrugge and Ascione reported that people are more likely to seek medical care when musculoskeletal symptoms compel restricted activity.[94] When symptoms occur in temporal association with work, the question usually arises as to whether the occupational exposure contributed to development of symptoms and/or an underlying disease process.

The purpose of this chapter is to discuss the multifactorial nature of neuromusculoskeletal conditions of the upper extremity and to demonstrate how dissimilar etiologic philosophies and clinical protocols can affect decisions regarding causation and disability. **Carpal tunnel syndrome** (CTS) is emphasized because it is the most well-known, objectively diagnosed condition included in the classification of neuromusculoskeletal disorders of the upper extremity.

The criteria considered (or not considered) during the diagnostic process may determine whether a neuromusculoskeletal condition of the upper extremity is ascribed to repetitive or forceful occupational exposure. If it is felt the symptoms are an ordinary life experience and not associated with work, determination of etiology generally is not of primary concern. If the symptoms are attributed to the physical nature of work, determination of etiology can become complex, and factors such as secondary gain and culpability may exert an influence. Szabo[88] stated that in managing a patient the clinician has four tasks, three of them medical and one bureaucratic. He said the physician's requirement to determine whether a condition is "caused" by the job is not a medical mandate but a bureaucratic one, since such a determination is "medically" impossible.[88] Harber and Shusterman suggested that societal decisions, not scientific method, must determine how much certainty is necessary to reach conclusions about the presence or absence of causal relationship.[42] In a patient management milieu that involves questions of causality, the physician must consider sometimes ambiguous factors that may involve not only unfamiliar areas of medical science, but areas that are outside the realm of medicine.

HISTORIC CONTEXT

Most serious observers agree that neuromusculoskeletal conditions exist in the workplace and that some of these occur at least in part as a result of occupational exposure. Some feel that repetitive occupational physical activity results in these conditions. Silverstein et al. reported CTS was strongly associated with high force–high repetition work in a group of 652 active workers,[80] and Hagberg et al. concluded that exposure to physical workload factors is probably a major risk factor for CTS in several types of worker populations.[38] Others feel that occupational activity is not generally a major factor. They cite other sources of causation, such as personal factors, psychosocial phenomena, and avocational stressors.[35,44,60,66,86,95] It is Hadler's opinion that most arm pain, whether inside or outside the workplace, is a predicament of life.[37] The medical validity of many conditions included within the category of work-related musculoskeletal disorders (Table 1) also has been questioned.[51,52,96]

In a review of the history of carpal tunnel syndrome, Amadio confirmed that in retrospect CTS was present and clinically observed in the final decades of the 19th century, although the true nature remained unknown and surgical treatment was not yet available.[1] In the early 20th century, some researchers reported occupational exposure to be responsible for complaints of the upper extremities. A condition resembling CTS was identified by Hunt and felt by him to be due to occupational overuse.[45] In 1920, Brouwer reported on 14 cases with features of thenar atrophy. He concluded that hyperfunction of the thumb played an etiologic role, but that this was an insufficient explanation. He opined that study of phylogenesis of involved muscles could elucidate issues of vulnerability for the development of the underlying disease.[14] Brouwer and other early researchers felt the thenar muscles were especially susceptible to degeneration as a result of trauma. (Later studies have shown thenar muscle wasting to indicate the presence of chronic slowing of the median nerve, as evidenced by involvement of the motor fibers,[73] and to be unrelated to trauma.) In 1947, Brain, Wright, and Wilkinson reported on a group of six females who underwent carpal tunnel release. They stated there could be little doubt that occupation was a causal factor for the carpal tunnel condition.[13]

These reports were countered by Phalen and Kendrick who in 1957 reported that spontaneous compression neuropathy of the median nerve in the carpal tunnel is not an occupational disease.[72] As the second half of the century progressed, CTS came to be acknowledged as occurring most often in middle-aged homemakers.[72,73,84,85] Stevens found that excessive hand use was an associated condition in only 5.9% of CTS cases.[85] Age, gender, pregnancy, and health problems such as diabetes, thyroid disease, rheumatoid arthritis, and obesity were found to be predisposing conditions for the development of median neuropathy and for CTS.[19,73,74,84,85,95]

TABLE 1. Classes of Upper Extremity Neuromusculoskeletal Conditions

A. Frequent Nonpathological Neuromusculoskeletal Conditions
These are part of life and usually resolve without medical intervention. No disability.

Aches and pains	Minor sprains and strains	Myofascial tightness
Fatigue	Swelling due to inactivity	Thermal discomfort
Stiffness	Sleepiness in extremity	

B. Frequently Diagnosed Pathological Neuromusculoskeletal Conditions
These are pathological and usually require medical intervention. Disability usually temporary.

Cubital tunnel syndrome	Severe sprains and strains	Carpal tunnel syndrome
Medial epicondylitis	DeQuervain's tenosynovitis	Lateral epicondylitis
Ganglia	Trigger Digits	Dupuytren's contracture
	Raynaud's disease	

C. Frequently Misdiagnosed Neuromusculoskeletal Conditions
These usually represent nonspecific discomfort misdiagnosed as disease. Minimal potential for physical disability. Potential for psychological disability if accurate diagnosis not obtained.

Flexor tenosynovitis	Thoracic outlet syndrome	Tendinitis
Hand/arm vibration syndrome	Reflex sympathetic dystrophy	Fibromyalgia

D. Nonspecifc Umbrella Terms With No Specific Objective Findings
These terms indicate a lack of diagnostic precision and objectivity. Used to describe subjective complaints. Potential for physical and psychological disability if accurate diagnosis not obtained.

Cumulative trauma disorders	Repetition strain injuries	Repetitive motion disorders
Repetitive motion injuries	Work-related musculoskeletal disorders	Overuse syndrome
Wear and tear disorders	Ergonomic disorders	

Proliferation of computers in the U.S. workplace in the 1980s coupled with awareness of an epidemic of "repetition strain injuries" in Australia[44,46] are cited by many as catalysts for a new round of research concerning the etiology of neuromusculoskeletal conditions of the upper extremities. Consistent with this, several factors led to the inclusion of work as a potential risk for these conditions. One was the advancement of alternative diagnostic criteria, which redefined injury and disease, resulting in a greater propensity for soft tissue discomfort to be elevated to a level of diagnostic significance.[41] Another factor in the increased prevalence of work-related upper extremity disorders was liberalization of a medicolegal system which offers monetary reward or other secondary gain to compensate for musculoskeletal conditions felt to result from work exposure. Introduction of mandatory employer-maintained OSHA logs for documentation of workplace incidents and subjective complaints of discomfort further enhanced a perception that the occurrence of upper extremity conditions in the workplace has escalated. Another factor is the anxiety-provoking reports generated by the lay press which advance the concept that an epidemic of debilitating injuries has stemmed from repetitive work tasks.

In "The Pain Perplex,"[29] author Gawande comments that some forms of chronic pain behave astonishingly like social epidemics. He recounts the well-known Australian epidemic of **repetitive strain injury** (RSI) in the 1980s, which primarily involved keyboard operators. The epidemic manifested itself in a sudden, dramatic outbreak of arm symptoms associated with keyboard use that progressed to a disabling status involving months of time loss from work. Diagnostic efforts suffered from a lack of objective findings, and clusters of affected workers appeared within single organizations and in disparate worksites involving the same and other occupations. The epidemic largely subsided—as suddenly as it began—by 1987. The life cycle of the Australian epidemic recounted by Gawande and reported by others[44,46] shares common features with other historic outbreaks of upper extremity complaints in which psychosocial aspects seemed to outweigh physiologic manifestations (Table 2). In likening the Australian outbreak to the current endemic of upper extremity complaints in the U.S. workplace, Gawande comments that salient risk factors seem to be social rather than physical, although he adds that the pain experience is real regardless of etiology, known or unknown. The convergence of these medical, bureaucratic, societal, and historic factors has coalesced in the form of an elevated focus on soft tissue discomfort of the upper extremities, leading to differing philosophies as to what constitutes injury or disease, and its cause.

THE TRADITIONAL MODEL

The traditional medical model (Fig. 1) maintains that objective evidence of injury or pathology must be demonstrated if neuromusculoskeletal conditions are to be considered diagnosable. This is **evidence-based medicine,** a generic term describing an approach to clinical practice that is systematic, objective, and as scientific as possible.[34] When this traditional model is adhered to, the prevalence of the upper extremity conditions diagnosed by physicians is generally limited. Appropriate treatment for cases of injury and disease identified under this model is usually not difficult to determine as it is based on the specific nature of the identified pathology. Prevention of neuromusculoskeletal conditions within this model also is generally a clearcut, objective process. The involved anatomic structures can be identified, and ergonomic and administrative interventions can be used to target those structures for reduction of force and repetition at the worksite. Any permanent impairment can be determined objectively following application of curative treatment to the diagnosed condition.

While this model is supported by the rigors of scientific and clinical methodology, it *does not account for the range of symptomatic experiences of humans in the workplace.* This limitation, in turn, drives research to understand the various pathways that can lead to the symptomatic experience, and it also has facilitated the emergence of an alternative model as to what constitutes injury or disease.

THE SYMPTOM-BASED MODEL

In the symptom-based model (see Fig. 1), soft tissue discomfort that would not achieve diagnostic status under the traditional medical model is considered to represent a diagnosable condition. This model does not require objective evidence of

TABLE 2.   Epidemics of Neuromusculoskeletal Conditions of the Upper Extremity

Location/ Industry	Condition	Years	Maximum Relative Claims Ratio	Comments
Japan/Clerical Workers[57]	Cervicobrachial disorder	1960–1973	33-fold (1965/1960)	Resolved with rest breaks; hence not pathological
United States/ Meat Packing[55]	Carpal tunnel release surgery	1971–1983	22.7-fold (Illinois/Iowa) 23-fold (1981/1971)	Surgery rates related to state compensation rates
Australia/ Telecom Australia[44]	Repetition strain injury	1981–1987	2.77-fold (Western Australia/New South Wales) 35.6-fold (1985/1981)	Resolved when compensation denied; hence, not pathological
United States/ U.S. West Telecom[35]	Cumulative trauma disorder	1988–1990	30-fold (Oregon/Utah)	Continues at dissimilar rates in different states

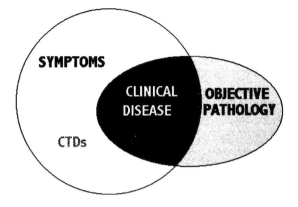

FIGURE 1. Comparison of the traditional model of disease and the symptom-based model. The circle represents symptoms. The ellipse represents objective pathology. The portion of the ellipse within the circle represents the area where diagnostic criteria for both models meet. The intersection of the circle and the ellipse (*black area*) indicates clinical disease, which is the focus of the traditional model. The focus of the symptom-based model is the entire circle, often referred to as cumulative trauma disorder (CTD), and includes symptoms both confirmed and unconfirmed by objective pathology. The gray area represents asymptomatic pathology, which may at some future date become symptomatic. There are more persons with symptoms (CTDs) than with objectively-confirmed clinical disease.

pathology for diagnosis. The exclusive use of subjective diagnostic criteria, i.e., symptoms, creates a greatly expanded prevalence of symptom-based conditions elevated to the level of "pathology." Under this model there is no clearly defined pathway to treatment, since specific tissue pathology generally is not identified. Symptoms essentially become the disease, creating a circumstance in which the goal of treatment is to palliate symptoms rather than to cure pathology.

The diagnosis of thoracic outlet syndrome (TOS) illustrates the impreciseness of symptom-based diagnostic methods.[77,98] Many patients receive a diagnosis of TOS based on the presence of ill-defined symptoms in the trunk and upper extremities and on general clinical impressions absent confirmatory tests which provide objective results. This has come to be termed *disputed* neurogenic TOS and has been said to have many similarities to the Australian RSI epidemic.[98] Wilbourn, a respected authority on the etiology and diagnosis of TOS, reports that there is little agreement not only with the diagnosis but with the methods used to develop the diagnosis. Wilbourn[97,98] states it is common for a given *disputed* TOS (diagnostic) procedure to be considered extremely useful by one proponent and worthless by another. Those who disagree suggest that technology is not yet refined enough to measure the complaints objectively and that congenital anomalies in the neck and thoracic outlet are common and "predispose" a large part of the general population to develop neurovascular symptoms that affect the upper extremities.[77] This lack of agreement among experts in the field points out the subjective nature and dearth of objective diagnostic information present within the symptom-based model for disease and injury.

Szabo states that under a model which implies presumptive etiology there are few comprehensive prospective studies, and reliable data are not available to guide the design for programs of treatment and rehabilitation.[88] Prevention of symptom-based conditions is also difficult to achieve because there is no requirement that a

pathologically involved soft tissue structure or structures be present to target for reduced exposure to force and/or repetition.

The emergence of the symptom-based model has sparked significant debate in jurisdictions concerned with workplace injuries and disease. In its suggestion that the traditional medical model of disease and injury is too narrow to address the problems of
today's workers, the symptom-based model has had significant socioeconomic impact.
In view of the growing acceptance of the symptom-based model of pathology it is useful to understand the evolution of the terminology upon which the concept is based.

Symptom-Based Diagnostic Terms

The symptom-based model of disease and injury has been presented in many
forms and refined as additional scientific evidence, both for and against it, became
available. The term *cumulative trauma disorder* was used as early as 1966,[91] and *repetition strain injury* was used widely in Australia in the 1970s and 1980s to describe
an outbreak of upper extremity complaints in telephonists and related occupations.[44,46] Within the symptom-based model, CTDs and RSIs have achieved a level of
common usage, even in a diagnostic sense. The term *work-related musculoskeletal
disorder* has emerged as the preferred nomenclature of governmental agencies such
as OSHA and NIOSH. *Repetitive motion disorders* (RMDs) constitute a special category of worker injury/illness in Bureau of Labor Statistics (BLS) reports.

The various "umbrella" terms describe nonspecific patterns of discomfort which
may lack objective evidence of pathologic involvement. When used for categorization
purposes they also can include upper extremity conditions with specific pathologic features, such as carpal tunnel syndrome, tendinitis, and deQuervain's. The nomenclature
itself often implies etiology in its linking of symptomatic complaints with the implicated activity. Armstrong stated that the term CTD was meant to reference a certain
class of disorders but was not intended to be used diagnostically.[4] A literature review
by Vender, Kasdan et al. suggests that CTD is not an accepted term within the scientific community.[93] In this review the authors analyze the epidemiological literature surrounding hypothesized work-related associations between various upper extremity
musculoskeletal disorders and alleged risk factors. They state that while many studies
have been conducted and articles written based on the assumption that the CTD hypothesis is factual, no definition of CTD has been agreed upon.[18,22,31,93]

In its initial drafts of a national ergonomic standard, OSHA used the term cumulative trauma disorder. This term implies that upper extremity neuromusculoskeletal
complaints in the workplace are caused by microtrauma inflicted over time. Computer
keyboard use is often considered to inflict cumulative trauma to the upper extremities,
which over time can be injurious, but this concept has not won support in the U.S.
Court systems.[3] The courts have been consistent in rendering opinions that the concept
of keyboard-related upper extremity conditions lack scientific merit and that plaintiffs
cannot prove injury from keyboard exposure. Researchers also have not succeeded in
demonstrating a dose-response relationship between repetitive work and the development of objectively confirmed upper extremity conditions. Two recent studies report
dose-response relationships between industrial exposure and symptoms, but neither
identifies a statistically significant link between repetition and objectively confirmed
nerve pathology.[7,50] Thus physicians determining etiology lack objective information
when asked to determine at what point keyboard use or other repetitive hand use constitutes hazard.[32,36] The ambiguity of the term coupled with the lack of scientific evidence for cumulative trauma occasioned a review of the term CTD, and subsequently
some proponents of the symptom-based model have substituted the term *work-related
musculoskeletal disorders* as described by Hales and Bernard.[41]

Researchers in this field have found flaws in the commonly accepted symptom-based nomenclature. Gerr et al. said that the nomenclature describing upper extremity musculoskeletal disorders of occupational origin is confusing and internally inconsistent. They point out that some terms refer to well-defined clinical entities and others are vague or inclusive of less well-defined soft tissue disorders.[31] Hagberg et al. blamed some of the confusion and controversy in occupational injury research to a lack of clearly defined terms and concepts, stating that the lack of consistent definitions creates a difficult challenge to even define a research question in occupational injury.[39]

Terminology aside, the focus of the symptom-based model remains that of ascribing causation based on temporal associations between symptoms and occupational exposure. In contrast, the focus of the traditional medical model of disease and injury remains that of ascribing causation when there is objective evidence of upper extremity pathology.

EVIDENCE FOR AND AGAINST OCCUPATIONAL ETIOLOGY

As with those engaged in recreational pursuits, some workers develop neuromusculoskeletal conditions of the upper extremities. According to the BLS and state workers' compensation statistics,[26,70] workers in different occupations report upper extremity complaints at different rates. As reported by the BLS, the incidence of reported RMDs increased from 0.3 cases/1000 workers in 1978 to 3.8 cases/1000 workers in 1993, and then declined slightly (1997) to 3.2 cases/1000 workers. Approximately 55% of these reported RMDs are hand/wrist disorders, with CTS predominating.

The BLS data suggest that rates of RMDs differ significantly by industry. Industries with primarily blue-collar workers (e.g., manufacturing) typically report the conditions at higher rates than industries with predominantly white-collar workers (e.g., business, insurance, and finance).[26,70] Differences in reported rates are interpreted by some, including government agencies, to indicate differences in actual rates and to demonstrate work-related etiology. The findings point toward an increased association between neuromusculoskeletal conditions and blue-collar jobs, but they do not consider the effect of intrinsic factors, lifestyle behaviors, and overall health status. The conditions are often reported after some precipitating physical event in conjunction with work or a recreational pursuit. In many cases, however, there are preexisting personal and lifestyle factors or underlying tissue pathology (e.g., peripheral nerve slowing) or susceptibility to pathology that predispose to the development of these conditions.[6,60,66,75,85]

Peer-Reviewed Literature is Divided

In spite of growing acceptance for the symptom-based model and the idea that these conditions are generally work-related, peer-reviewed literature on the subject remains divided. The literature contains case reports and cross-sectional studies that link self-reported symptoms to self-reported ergonomic hazard exposure.[8,41,54,68] Some studies link objectively confirmed medical diagnoses to self-reported ergonomic hazard exposure[24] or self-reported symptoms to objectively measured ergonomic hazard exposure.[80] Arguments based on biological plausibility abound,[8,41,54,68] and inconsistencies are explained as examples of selection bias or survivor bias.[8,17,38,41,68,81]

Reviews of the literature concerning relationships between repetitive work exposure and neuromusculoskeletal conditions of the upper extremities reveal that most studies interpreted to show a significant, positive relationship lack specific criteria for validity.[8,56,86,93] Gerr et al. stated that much of the literature examining the relationships of upper-extremity musculoskeletal health outcomes to occupational factors is flawed. They found few such studies to have employed rigorous assessments of exposure or well-defined objective measures of outcomes.[31] Current scrutiny of the pioneering study of Brain et al. reveals that it lacked support for the conclusion that occupation is a causative factor for CTS.[13] Five of the six middle-aged female patients (average age 55) in the study were housewives, and the sixth patient, a tailoress, was reported to have a history of hand trauma unrelated to her employment. All six patients presented with thenar atrophy, which is now known to be a manifestation of a chronic neuropathic process and not the result of recent trauma or unaccustomed hand use, as reported by the authors. The article suggests that the authors considered wartime housekeeping to be an occupation, which could further confuse efforts to differentiate between occupational hand use and the activities of daily living.

It also has been pointed out that the literature lacks prospective, longitudinal studies that demonstrate a consistent, positive relationship between *objective* measures of repetitive work exposure and objectively confirmed diagnoses.[32,56,94] Cross-sectional studies cannot demonstrate causation; they can only generate hypotheses to be tested.[36,56] Longitudinal studies, in contrast, can give the critical dimension of time, which allows demonstration that cause preceded effect, and that there is a consistent, time-dependent dose effect.

To date there are no peer-reviewed longitudinal studies that confirm statistically significant, independent, positive relationships between work and the development of neuromusculoskeletal conditions of the upper extremities. A recent longitudinal study of risk factors for neck and upper limb disorders, from Sweden, fails to isolate specific work factors as a primary cause for hand and wrist conditions. The authors state that their findings may point to psychosocial factors (total overload and dissatisfaction with life as a whole) as critical to development of upper extremity disorders.[27]

In addition to excluding consideration of psychosocial factors, much of the literature has failed to consider personal and lifestyle factors (Table 3) such as heredity, age, gender, race, height, weight, body mass index, avocational activities, medical history, use of legal drugs, general health, and mental health, which, along with other factors, have been shown to be significant risk factors for the conditions in question.[6,19–21,23,58–67,72–75,84,85,87,89,90,93,95]

In the case of CTS, the more specific the diagnosis and the longer the time interval of the study, the less likely is a consistent, positive relationship with work factors to be found.[36,58–67] CTS is an appropriate example to introduce into a discussion of the etiology of neuromusculoskeletal conditions of the upper extremity since it is commonly cited as exemplifying the many conditions included under the umbrella of the symptom-based model. It involves a diagnosis based on specific clinical findings, and it is confirmed objectively by the presence of organic nerve pathology. In a prospective longitudinal study of CTS that employed an objective case definition, we found no significant role for repetitive or forceful work exposure in predicting future hand/wrist symptoms and CTS.[59] In contrast, initial personal and lifestyle factors classified hands by future CTS status, demonstrating the often and overlooked pre-eminent role of intrinsic factors in the etiology of CTS.[58–67] In 1997, Moore and Prezzia applied, to a selected group of articles on CTS etiology, nine criteria used in the scientific community to evaluate epidemiologic studies to determine if reported or postulated associations are causal.[56] Based on their findings, they stated that it is currently not possible to conclude that work *causes* carpal tunnel syndrome. Among findings in the reviewed articles were lack of consistency of association between studies and no dose relationship between work exposure and CTS.

Our longitudinal study of CTS referenced above suggests that the net independent effect of work is beneficial, not harmful.[58–67] This meshes with a hypothesis ad-

TABLE 3.   Risk Factors Associated with Carpal Tunnel Syndrome

Risk Factor	References

1. Family History
  a) autosomal dominant
  b) amyloidosis
  c) connective tissue disorders
  d) mesenchymal syndrome
	Bonnici (10), Gossett (33), Nathan (66), Radecki (75)

2. Older Age	Nathan (66), Phalen (73,74), Radecki (75), Seror (79), Stevens (84)

3. Female Gender
  a) homemakers
  b) perimenopausal
	Phalen (73,74), Radecki (75), Seror (79), Stevens (84,85), Vessey (95)

4. White Race	(Nathan (66), Radecki (75), Tanaka (89)
5. Obesity	DeKrom (20), Nathan (58), Radecki (75), Vessey (95)

6. Wrist Dimensions
  a) deeper wrists
  b) squarer wrists
	Latko (50), Nathan (58,66), Radecki (75)

7. Lack of Aerobic Exercise	Nathan (60,66)
8. Tobacco Use	Nathan (65,66), Vessey (95)
9. Alcohol Abuse/Nonuse	Cseuz (19), Nathan (65,66), Phalen (73)
10. Diabetes Mellitus	Atcheson (6), Phalen (73,74), Stevens (85)
11. Thyroid Disease	Phalen (73,74), Stevens (85)
12. Rheumatoid Disease	Atcheson (6), Phalen (73,74), Stevens (85)
13. Pregnancy	Phalen (73,74), Radecki (75), Stevens (85)
14. Gout	Phalen (73,74)
15. Trauma (acute)	Phalen (73,74), Stevens (85)
16. Hypertension	Nathan (66), Radecki (75)

vanced by Ross and Mirowsky[78] that various aspects surrounding full-time employment keep workers healthy. Compared to homemaking, unemployment, part-time employment, or retirement, the authors found full-time employment to be associated with the best overall health status and the slowest deterioration in health status.[78] We and others have found that lifestyle and health habits matter. Those who smoke cigarettes and those who abuse alcohol are more likely to develop neuromusculoskeletal conditions of the upper extremities.[16,19,65,66,95] This is consistent with literature that links poor health habits to a significantly greater incidence of medical conditions such as heart disease, high blood pressure, and diabetes.[71,87] In contrast, we have observed workers, in a large variety of physically challenging occupations, who have remained healthy after 20 or more years of consecutive occupational exposure.[59,67] We also have observed workers reporting symptoms and having objective evidence of upper extremity conditions after less than a week on the job.

These observations suggest that most work activities are not harmful for most workers, in terms of development of CTS, and that factors outside of work exposure are influential to the development of CTS and other conditions classified as neuromusculoskeletal conditions of the upper extremities. In our observations we have found that most workers who perform similar tasks do not develop similar symptoms or develop no symptoms at all. This erodes a concept of consistent work relationships and mandates consideration of conditions other than the worksite for the development of neuromusculoskeletal complaints of the upper extremities.

Armstrong and co-researchers[5] developed a conceptual model for work-related neck and upper-limb musculoskeletal disorders. The model predicted that the human neuromusculoskeletal system can be overloaded by physical requirements of the job, resulting in "microfailures" which over time cascade into "macrofailures" and manifest clinically as symptoms and disease. This model allows that the ability to adapt to physical stresses may differ among individuals, but the main concern expressed by Armstrong, et al. was of an imbalance between work stresses and the ability of workers to adapt to the work. The work stresses were viewed as primary and modifiable and, therefore, culpable and compensable in the medicolegal system. The model did not account for the knowledge that living tissue responds positively to stress by remodeling and regenerating to a form that has a greater tolerance for mechanical stress.[28] Thus, it could be postulated that physical stresses associated with repetitive activity, continued over time, can increase, rather than decrease, tolerance for repetitive motion. This is consistent with findings from a retrospective cohort study of 484 men and women aged 41–58 years by Torgen et al. This study suggests that a physically heavy workload has a possible maintaining and/or training effect of the upper extremities.[92]

VARIATIONS IN TREATMENT METHODS

In spite of rather striking differences between the traditional model of disease and injury and the symptom-based model, the goal of each is to reduce discomfort and to enhance workplace productivity. The pathways toward this goal are influenced by the model that is embraced. In the most general sense, determinations as to whether these conditions are considered work related depends on one's perspective as to which category carries the greater weight of causation: predisposing personal factors or precipitating physical events. Among physicians the determination might be based on personal values, anecdotal experiences, or philosophical issues. In this atmosphere it is unlikely that agreement as to causation will occur any time soon. Thus we are left to try to resolve these dilemmas through our best intuitive "guess" and through interpretation of a body of literature that is deeply polarized and lacks consensus. In the final application, issues of etiology are often determined through an adversarial medicolegal process. This can exact significant monetary and personal cost from both worker and employer and frustration from physicians not trained for the task of medical adjudication. The prevalence of this less-than-satisfactory form of retrospective dispute resolution points out the necessity for emphasis on prospective workplace health and wellness programs, functional capacities screening, ergonomic intervention, engineering changes, and effective medical management.

Treatment within the traditional model is generally straightforward. Pathologically involved structures are identified and diagnosed, and the nature of the pathology is determined. Treatment protocol can be formulated to address specific pathologically involved structures. Ergonomic intervention strategies within this model also are rather well defined. Once a pathologically involved structure is identified, it can usually be determined if job-related biomechanical forces have influenced development of the condition. If there is a correlation, specific engineering, ergonomic, and administrative steps can be exercised to reduce force and repetition loads on the involved anatomic structures, or workers can be reassigned to tasks that they are physically capable of performing.

Within the framework of the symptom-based model, treatment and intervention strategies are less well defined. Because there is frequently no definable pathology or clearly identified anatomic involvement, it is difficult to formulate an objectively justifiable treatment plan. Treatment and intervention strategies under the symptom-based model often are limited to recommendations for a general and nonspecific decrease in workload, or work cessation.[41,54] This approach can be useful in short-term symptom management, but can lead to the presumption of disability rather than enabling full and sustained return to employment.

Many conditions identified under both the traditional and symptom-based models are associated with **poor health habits** and **compromised levels of physical fitness.** We believe much can be done to alleviate these associated conditions and to limit the magnitude of symptom-based neuromusculoskeletal conditions that present in the workplace. Since basic health and fitness issues are at the heart of many conditions, it is reasonable that employer-sponsored treatment and intervention strategies should include comprehensive health education programs that focus on weight loss, smoking cessation, and sound nutritional principles.

Low levels of physical fitness are often associated with the development of neuromusculoskeletal conditions of the upper extremities. Because of this association, a program of regular conditioning exercises also should be encouraged. Recent data in the area of industrial physical conditioning is lacking, but it is reasonable to expect that an employer-sponsored program of conditioning and flexibility exercises could prove cost effective in the management of many soft tissue-musculoskeletal symptom complexes included in the classification of work-related neuromusculoskeletal disorders. Such is the experience reported by Ethicon, Inc. In the early 1980s, Ethicon established an onsite exercise program as one component of a far-reaching ergonomics program.[53] After more than 5 years of experience with the exercise program, it was determined that the exercises, used intermittently during the work day, conferred both physiologic and psychologic benefit for the employees. As with Ethicon, other employers may find that resources for programs of health education and fitness will garner financial and productivity benefits which greatly exceed those associated with intervention through work modification for work cessation.

An employee selection process incorporating functional capacity tests can also be an effective preventative tool, so long as it addresses Americans With Disabilities Act (ADA) concerns and conforms to applicable governmental nondiscrimination laws. Many employers have demonstrated that physically matching the employee to the job yields greater benefits to both employer and employee than more costly attempts to match (modify) the job to fit the worker.[9,40,43] Functional capacity testing is suited particularly to occupations which involve heavy physical workload.

DETERMINING IMPAIRMENT OF THE UPPER EXTREMITIES

Even the most vigorous attempts at treatment and prevention cannot successfully target every component of neuromusculoskeletal conditions felt to interfere significantly with physical performance and job function. For those cases, **quantification of impairment** must be addressed.

Within the traditional model of pathology-based disease and injury, impairment of the upper extremities can be determined on an objective basis. The impairment is most often proportional to the degree of residual pathologic involvement in the neuromusculoskeletal structures. An example of this approach is the process involved in assessing impairment from a traumatically amputated digit. The nature and extent of the residual pathology can be measured. The disability rating is then accomplished by comparing the objectively measured pathology with tables of impairment generated by the American Medical Association.[2] The result is an impairment rating based on objective principles. This can be interpreted accurately by insurance administrators and reproduced by other examiners with similar experience in disability rating.

Where neuromusculoskeletal conditions have been identified under the symptom-based model, rating of impairment is much less straightforward. There is often no objective evidence of pathology upon which to base assessment of impairment or disability. The individual who has only subjective complaints of activity/work intolerance, and no evidence of upper extremity pathology, is much more challenging to assess for determination of impairment. Symptoms by themselves do not constitute a ratable impairment, and there may be a wide range of opinions regarding the degree of impairment that results from the reported work intolerance. Such impairment ratings are rarely reproducible by others involved in developing permanent impairment ratings. The impairment is likely to be specific only to certain work tasks and work demand levels, and often results, at least in part, from underlying intrinsic health issues or a compromised state of physical fitness. Disability in this model is a situational and impermanent circumstance, which may fluctuate over time.

CONCLUSION

Review of the body of literature suggests that the majority of workers in most occupations remain healthy and physically capable of performing work tasks. In studies that demonstrate associations between work exposure and the development of upper extremity disorders, only a fraction of the exposed workers were classified as having acquired a neuromusculoskeletal condition of the upper extremity.[25–27,69,80] A work and health association is supported by Ross and Mirowsky's[78] finding that persons who remain in full-time employment are more healthy than those who are unemployed or employed only part-time. From this, researchers involved in investigations of the upper extremities might hypothesize that, in part, individuals remain physically capable of vocational activities because they are engaged in vocational activities that promote (by maintaining) a consistent level of physical conditioning specific to the required tasks.

It is the fraction of workers who develop neuromusculoskeletal problems of the upper extremities who are of concern to physicians engaged in making decisions concerning diagnosis, causation, and disability. So long as there are philosophical and jurisdictional differences in the approach to defining the conditions, and a lack of clearly defined terms and concepts, the field cannot achieve consensus. The workplace is dynamic in terms of modernization, automation, and composition of the workforce. During the war effort in the 1940s, females dominated the defense workforce, competing in typical male occupations. At the end of World War II large numbers of females returned to the traditional homemaker role, with males again dominating in the industrial setting. Census data reveal that in 1940 females made up 25% of the U.S. workforce. With the exception of the brief heightened work presence of females in the mid-1940s, female employment increased gradually over the decades. By 1997 nearly 50% of the total U.S. workforce was composed of females.[83] This points out dissimilarities in gender distributions between the current workforce and the workforce of 30 years ago. Such inconsistencies in historic workplace variables frustrate efforts to apply historic data to resolving the problems in today's workplace.

Those concerned with issues of causation of neuromusculoskeletal conditions of the upper extremity today (NIOSH, OSHA, ergonomists, employers, industry representatives, and attorneys) have deeply vested special interests and opposing and often adversarial philosophies. Within this complex maze, clinical considerations can be overshadowed by political and philosophical issues. In this circumstance the most effective strategy for the physician determining causation is one of detached clinical pragmatism. As clinicians, we have a general understanding of the degree and type of physical stresses required to cause pathologic involvement of soft tissue structures. The basic human tolerance to withstand resistive and repetitive activities has not changed through the years, even though the language and philosophical parameters describing the physiologic response to activity have evolved significantly.

In circumstances where emotionally charged issues concerning causation and compensability can be set aside, there is clearer recognition that certain forms of diagnosable neuromusculoskeletal conditions and a wide range of neuromusculoskeletal discomfort are present in the workplace. It seems reasonable that workers who experience neuromusculoskeletal discomfort while performing manual work will be less productive. These workers, because of discomfort they associate with work, may develop apprehension and hostility toward the work environment, and this can accelerate into negative outcomes for both employee and employer.

Physicians engaged in occupational medicine possess a wide variety of tools and techniques with the potential to prevent or significantly limit negative outcomes from these symptoms and conditions. Concern over issues of causation and culpability are critical factors that can inhibit implementation of available solutions. Rather than act as agents for blame-placing agencies, the occupational physician's chosen role should be that of managing physical problems when they present in the workplace, without having to exert concern for secondary and complicating issues of culpability and compensation. The design of current adjudicative systems, however, forces the occupational physician into a more complex role, and issues of culpability and compensation often must be addressed. When we believe the physical requirements of work have exceeded the worker's physical capacity and resulted in injury, we should be straightforward in stating the work was a significant contributing factor. If we find the physical requirements of the job have not exceeded the physiologic and structural limits of musculotendinous structures, we should feel justified in stating that the workplace is not a causative factor, despite popular opinion or prevailing attitudes.

By the scientific nature of our education and training we are required to understand and adhere to objective principles of anatomy and physiology. Opinions regarding etiology of neuromusculoskeletal conditions of the upper extremities should be based on the objective principles of anatomy and physiology and not be influenced by "convenience" labels which infer causation, unproven claims of epidemics of "repetitive motion disorders," or the shrill arguments of partisan "scientists" who posit that occupational activity, in general, is either harmful or protective, without obtaining detailed knowledge of the specific nature of work activities as they apply to the individual worker. As stated by Hadler, ". . . we must return the old common sense."[37] By applying a common sense approach to each worker's problem, we can override the fluctuating currents of philosophic thought and avoid reacting to sweeping statistical, philosophic, and partisan generalizations. The question of whether neuromusculoskeletal conditions of the upper extremity are work related can be addressed most effectively by analysis of the specific nature of work tasks in conjunction with analysis of the physical, medical, psychologic, and physiologic composition of the worker and analysis of the worker's lifestyle habits.

In a discussion of heuristic approaches to determining medical causation, Harber and Shusterman said that formal mathematical analysis using methods such as epidemiology, formal logic, and decision theory can provide considerable insight.[42] Within the scientific research environment it is possible to collect data on relative risks and to make predictive statements as to which workers are most likely to develop CTS or other neuromusculoskeletal conditions of the upper extremity. Care needs to be taken in extrapolating this information to determining causation at the level of the individual worker. Generalizations based on assessment of relative risks and statistical trends, while adequate for summarizing the large population experience, may contain information, which when applied at the individual level, could result in erroneous determinations as to causation.

The workplace and the worker form a nucleus for the study of occupational medicine. They are intertwined with the dynamics of change in the industrial, medical, and social environments. The effective occupationally oriented physician will move outside the confines of the workplace to gain a true and complete understanding of the universe of factors that weigh together to result in presentation of neuromusculoskeletal conditions of the upper extremity.

REFERENCES

1. Amadio PC: Historical review. The Mayo Clinic and carpal tunnel syndrome. Mayo Clin Proc 67:42–48, 1992.
2. American Medical Association. Guides to the Evaluation of Permanent Impairment, 4th edition. Chicago, AMA, 1993.
3. Anonymous: N.Y. jury rejects keyboard liability in DEC case. CTD News 7(7):1, 1997.
4. Armstrong TJ: Introduction to occupational disorders of the upper extremities. In: Occupational Disorders of the Upper Extremities. Ann Arbor, MI, Center for Occupational Health, Safety, and Engineering, 1990.
5. Armstrong TJ, Buckle P, Fine LJ, et al: A conceptual model for work-related neck and upper-limb musculoskeletal disorders. Scand J Work Environ Health 19:73–84, 1993.
6. Atcheson SG, Ward JR, Lowe W: Concurrent medical disease in work-related carpal tunnel syndrome. Arch Intern Med 158:1506–1512, 1998.
7. Atroshi I, Gummesson C, Johnsson R, et al: Prevalence of carpal tunnel syndrome in a general population. JAMA 282:153–158, 1999.
8. Bernard, et al: Musculoskeletal Disorders and Workplace Factors. A critical review of epidemiologic evidence for work-related musculoskeletal disorders of the neck, upper extremity, and back, 2nd printing. USDHHS, PHS. July 1997, DHHS (NIOSH) Publication No. 97-141.
9. Blankenship KL: Functional capacity evaluation (FCE) process, explanation of frequency, and physical demand levels by dot manual. In Blankenship KL: Industrial Rehabilitation I. A Seminar Syllabus. American Therapeutics, Inc, 1990, pp 2.01–2.12, 12.64, and 12.65.
10. Bonnici AV, Birjandi F, Spencer JD, et al: Chromosomal abnormalities in Dupuytren's contracture and carpal tunnel syndrome. J Hand Surg 17B:349–355, 1992.
11. Bonzani PJ, Millender L, Keelan B, Mangieri MG: Factors prolonging disability in work-related cumulative trauma disorders. J Hand Surg 22A:30–34, 1997.
12. Bortz WM II: Disuse and aging. JAMA 248:1203–1208, 1982.
13. Brain WR, Wright AD, Wilkinson M: Spontaneous compression of both median nerves in the carpal tunnel. Six cases treated surgically. The Lancet 1:277–282, March 1947.
14. Brouwer B: The significance of phylogenic and ontogenic studies for the neuropathologist. J Nerv Mental Dis 51:113–136, 1920.
15. Brown PW: The role of motivation in the recovery of the hand. In Kasdan ML (ed): Occupational Hand & Upper Extremity Injuries & Diseases, 2nd ed. Philadelphia, Hanley & Belfus, 1997, pp 5–14.
16. Burge P, Hoy G, Regan P, Miline R: Smoking, alcohol, and the risk of Dupuytren's contracture. J Bone Joint Surg 79B:206–210, 1997.
17. Cannon LJ, Bernacki EJ, Walter SD: Personal and occupational factors associated with carpal tunnel syndrome. J Occup Med 23:255–258, 1981.
18. CDC-NIOSH: Cumulative Trauman Disorders in the Workplace. Bibliography. USDHHS, PHS. 1995. DHHS (NIOSH) Publ No. 95–119.
19. Cseuz KA, Thomas JE, Lambert EH, et al: Long-term results of operation for carpal tunnel syndrome. Mayo Clin Proc 41:232–241, 1966.
20. DeKrom MCTFM, Kester ADM, Knipschild PG, Spaans F: Risk factors for carpal tunnel syndrome. Am J Epidemiol 132:1021–1110, 1990.
21. Derebery VJ: Etiologies and prevalence of occupational upper extremity injuries. In Kasdan ML (ed): Occupational Hand & Upper Extremity Injuries & Diseases, 2nd ed. Philadelphia, Hanley & Belfus, 1997, pp 49–58.
22. Dobyns JH: Cumulative trauma disorder of the upper limb. Hand Clinics 7:587–595, 1991.
23. Dzwierzynski WW, Grunert BK, Rusch MD, et al: Psychometric assessment of patients with chronic upper extremity pain attributed to workplace exposure. J Hand Surg 24A:46–52, 1999.
24. English CJ, Maclaren WM, et al: Relations between upper limb soft tissue disorders and repetitive movements at work. Am J Indust Med 27:75–90, 1995.
25. Feldman RG, Travers PH, Chirico-Post J, Keyserling WM: Risk assessment in electronic assembly workers: Carpal tunnel syndrome. J Hand Surg 12A:849–855, 1987.
26. Franklin GM, Haug J, Heyer N, et al: Occupational carpal tunnel syndrome in Washington State, 1984–1988. Am J Public Health 81:741–746, 1991.

27. Fredriksson K, Alfredsson L, Koster M, et al: Risk factors for neck and upper limb disorders: Results from 24 years of follow-up. Occup Environ Med 56:59–66, 1999.

28. Frost HM: Skeletal structural adaptations to mechanical usage: Mechanical influences on intact fibrous tissue. Anat Record 226:433–439, 1990.

29. Gawande A: The pain perplex. A new theory is revising the centuries-old model of how we feel pain. New Yorker September 21, 1998, pp 86–91.

30. Gemme G: Diagnostics of hand-arm system disorders in workers who use vibrating tools. Occup Environ Med 54:90–95, 1997.

31. Gerr F, Letz R, Landrigan PJ: Upper-extremity musculoskeletal disorders of occupational origin. Ann Rev Publ Health 12:543–566, 1991.

32. Gerr F, Marcus M, Ortiz DJ: Methodological limitations in the study of video display terminal use and upper extremity musculoskeletal disorders. Am J Indust Med 29:649–656, 1996.

33. Gossett JG, Chance PF: Is there a familial carpal tunnel syndrome? An evaluation and literature review. Muscle Nerve 21:1533–1536, 1998.

34. Gots RE: Evidence-based medicine and the independent medical examiner. Hippocrates Lantern 6(2):17–21, 1999.

35. Hadler NM: Arm pain in the workplace. A small area analysis. J Occup Med 34:113–119, 1992.

36. Hadler NM: Repetitive upper-extremity motions in the workplace are not hazardous. J Hand Surg 22A:19–29, 1997.

37. Hadler NM: Carpal tunnel syndrome, diagnostic conundrum. Editorial. J Rheumatol 24:417–419, 1997.

38. Hagberg M, Morgenstern H, Kelsh M: Impact of occupations and job tasks on the prevalence of carpal tunnel syndrome. Scand J Work Environ Health 18:337–345, 1992.

39. Hagberg M, Chritiani D, Courtney TK, et al: Conceptual and definitional issues in occupational injury epidemiology. Am J Indust Med 32:106–115, 1997.

40. Hainer BL: Preplacement evaluations. Prim Care 21:237–247, 1994.

41. Hales TR, Bernard BP: Epidemiology of work-related musculoskeletal disorders. Orthop Clin NA 27:679–709, 1996.

42. Harber P, Shusterman D: Medical causation analysis heuristics. J Occup Environ Med 38:577–586, 1996.

43. Hart DL, Isernhagen SJ, Matheson LN: Guidelines for functional capacity evaluation of people with medical conditions. J Orthop Sports Phys Ther 18:682–686, 1993.

44. Hocking B: Epidemiological aspects of "repetition strain injury" in Telecom Australia. Med J Austral 147:218–222, 1987.

45. Hunt JR: The thenar and hypothenar types of neural atrophy of the hand. Am J Med Sci 141:224–241, 1911.

46. Ireland DCR: Repetition strain injury. The Australian experience—1992 update. J Hand Surg 20A:S53–S56, 1995.

47. Jablecki CK, Andary MT, So YT, et al: Literature review of the usefulness of nerve conduction studies and electromyography for the evaluation of patients with carpal tunnel syndrome. Muscle Nerve 16:1392–1414, 1993.

48. Kasdan ML: Preface to second edition. In Kasdan ML (ed): Occupational Hand & Upper Extremity Injuries & Diseases, 2nd ed. Philadelphia, Hanley & Belfus, 1997.

49. Katz JN, Larson MG, Fossel AH, Liang MH: Validation of a surveillance case definition of carpal tunnel syndrome. Am J Public Health 81:189–193, 1991.

50. Latko WA, Armstrong TJ, Franzblau A, et al: Cross-sectional study of the relationship between repetitive work and the prevalence of upper limb musculoskeletal disorders. Am J Indust Med 36:248–259, 1999.

51. Lister GD: Ergonomic disorders. Editorial. J Hand Surg 20A:353, 1995.

52. Louis DS: Are we there yet? Presidential address. J Hand Surg 23A:191–195, 1998.

53. Lutz G, Hansford T: Cumulative trauma disorder controls: The ergonomics program at Ethicon, Inc. J Hand Surg 12A:863–866, 1987.

54. Mackinnon SE, Novak CB: Clinical Perspective. Repetitive strain in the workplace. J Hand Surg 2–18, 1997.

55. Masear VR, Hayes JM, Hyde AG: An industrial cause of carpel tunnel syndrome. J Hand Surg 11A:222–227, 1986.

56. Moore JS, Prezzia C: Considerations in determining the work-relatedness of carpal tunnel syndrome. In Erdil M, Dickerson OB (eds): Cumulative Trauma Disorders: Prevention, Evaluation, and Treatment. New York, Van Nostrand Reinhold, 1997, pp 59–97.

57. Nakaseko M: Cases of occupational cervicobrachial disorder in Nippon Telephone and Telegraph. Personal communication as reported by Dr. Hocking (see ref. 44).

58. Nathan PA, Keniston RC, Myers LD, Meadows KD: Obesity as a risk factor for slowing of sensory conduction of the median nerve in industry. A cross-sectional and longitudinal study involving 429 workers. J Occup Med 34:379–383, 1992.

59. Nathan PA, Keniston RC, Myers LD, Meadows KD: Longitudinal study of median nerve sensory conduction in industry: Relationship to age, gender, hand dominance, occupational hand use, and clinical diagnosis. J Hand Surg 17A:850–857, 1992.

60. Nathan PA, Keniston RC: Carpal tunnel syndrome and its relation to general physical condition. Hand Clinics 9:253–261, 1993.

61. Nathan PA, Keniston RC, Meadows KD: Carpal tunnel syndrome in the workplace. Hippocrates' Lantern 2(2):1–5, 1993.

62. Nathan PA, Meadows KD, Keniston RC: Rehabilitation of carpal tunnel surgery patients using a short surgical incision and early program of physical therapy. J Hand Surg 18A: 1044–1050, 1993.

63. Nathan PA, Keniston RC, Meadows KD, Lockwood RS: Nerve conduction studies and carpal tunnel syndrome. Am J Indust Med 27:311–312, 1995.

64. Nathan PA, Keniston RC, Meadows KD: Carpal tunnel syndrome claims. In The Insurer's Handbook of Psychological Injury Claims. Seattle, Claims Books, 1995, pp 265–276.

65. Nathan PA, Keniston RC, Meadows KD, Lockwood RS: Tobacco, caffeine, alcohol, and carpal tunnel syndrome in American industry. J Occup Environ Med 38:290–298, 1996.

66. Nathan PA, Keniston RC: Carpal tunnel syndrome: Personal risk profile and role of intrinsic and behavioral factors. In Kasdan ML (ed): Occupational Hand & Upper Extremity Injuries & Diseases, 2nd ed. Philadelphia, Hanley & Belfus, 1997, pp. 129–139.

67. Nathan PA, Keniston RC, Myers LD, et al: Natural history of median nerve sensory conduction in industry: Relationship to symptoms and carpal tunnel syndrome in 558 hands over 11 years. Muscle Nerve 21:711–721, 1998.

68. National Research Council: Work-Related Musculoskeletal Disorders. Report, workshop summary, and workshop reports. Washington, DC, National Academy Press, 1999.

69. Nilsson T, Hagberg M, Burstrom L, Lundstrom R: A five-year follow-up of nerve conduction over the carpal tunnel. Arbette Och Halsa betensklaplig skriftserie. 5:117–120, 1995.

70. Oregon Department of Insurance and Finance and Oregon Department of Business and Consumer Services, Research and Analysis Section, Carpal Tunnel Syndrome in Oregon, 1984–1988, 1987–1991, 1990–1994, 1991–1995, 1996, 1997.

71. Pate RR, Pratt M, Blair SN, et al: Physical activity and public health. A recommendation from the Centers for Disease Control and Prevention and the American College of Sports Medicine. JAMA 273: 402–407, 1995.

72. Phalen GS, Kendrick JI: Compression neuropathy of the median nerve in the carpal tunnel. JAMA 164:524–530, 1957.

73. Phalen GS: The carpal tunnel syndrome: 17 years experience in diagnosis and treatment of 654 hands. J Bone Joint Surg 48A:211–228, 1966.

74. Phalen GS: The carpal tunnel syndrome. Clinical evaluation of 598 hands. Clin Orthop Rel Res 83:29–40, 1972.

75. Radecki P: Carpal tunnel syndrome. Effects of personal factors and associated medical conditions. Phys Med Rehabil Clin NA 8:419–437, 1997.

76. Rempel D, Evanoff B, Amadio PC, et al: Consensus criteria for the classification of carpal tunnel syndrome in epidemiologic studies. Am J Public Health 88:1447–1451, 1998.

77. Roos DB: Thoracic outlet syndrome is underdiagnosed. Muscle Nerve 22:126–129, 1999.

78. Ross CE, Mirowsky J: Does employment affect health? J Health Social Behavior 36:230–243, 1995.

79. Seror P, Nathan PA: Relative frequency of nerve conduction abnormalities at carpal tunnel and cubital tunnel in France and the United States. Importance of silent neuropathies and role of ulnar neuropathy after unsuccessful carpal tunnel syndrome release. Ann Chir Main 12:281–285, 1993.

80. Silverstein BA, Fine LJ, Armstrong TJ: Occupational factors and carpal tunnel syndrome. Am J Indust Med 11:343–358, 1987.

81. Silverstein B, Fine L, Stetson D: Hand-wrist disorders among investment casting plant workers. J Hand Surg 12A:838–844, 1987.

82. Silverstein BA, Armstrong TJ, Longmate A, Woody D: Can in-plant exercise control musculoskeletal symptoms? J Occup Med 30:922–927, 1988.

83. Smith KE, Bachu A: Women's labor force attachment patterns and maternity leave: A review of the literature. Population Division Working Paper No. 32. Washington, DC, Population Division, U.S. Bureau of the Census, Jan 1999.

84. Stevens JC, Beard CM, O'Fallon WM, et al: Carpal tunnel syndrome in Rochester, Minnesota, 1961 to 1980. Neurol 38:134–138, 1988.

85. Stevens JC, Beard CM, O'Fallon WM, et al: Conditions associated with carpal tunnel syndrome. Mayo Clin Proc 67:541–548, 1992.

86. Stock SR: Workplace ergonomic factors and the development of musculoskeletal disorders of the neck and upper extremity: A meta-analysis. Am J Indust Med 19:87–107, 1991.

87. Surgeon General's Report on Nutrition and Health: Coronary heart disease; high blood pressure; diabetes; obesity; skeletal diseases. Washington, DC, US Department of Health and Human Services, Public Health Service, 1988, pp 83–343.
88. Szabo RM: Overview. In Gordon SL, Blair SJ, Fine LJ (eds): Repetitive Motion Disorders of the Upper Extremity. Rosemont, IL, Am Acad Orthop Surg, 1995, p 419.
89. Tanaka S, Wild DK, Seligman PJ, et al: Prevalence and work-relatedness of self-reported carpal tunnel syndrome among U.S. workers: Analysis of the occupational health supplement data of 1988 National Health Interview Survery. Am J Indust Med 27:451–470, 1995.
90. Tanzer RC: The carpal tunnel syndrome. A clinical and anatomic study. J Bone Joint Surg 41A:626–634, 1959.
91. Tischuer ER: Some aspects of stress on forearm and hand in industry. J Occup Med 8:63–71, 1966.
92. Torgen M, Punnett L, Alfredsson L, Kilbom A: Physical capacity in relation to present and past physical load at work: A study of 484 men and women aged 41 to 58 years. Am J Indust Med 36:388–400, 1999.
93. Vender MI, Kasdan ML, Truppa KL: Upper extremity disorders: A literature review to determine work-relatedness. J Hand Surg 20A:534–541, 1995.
94. Verbrugge LM, Ascione FJ: Exploring the iceberg. Common symptoms and how people care for them. Medical Care 25:539–569, 1987.
95. Vessey MP, Villard-MacIntosh L, Yeates D: Epidemiology of carpal tunnel syndrome in women of childbearing age. Findings in a large cohort study. Int J Epidemiol 19:655–659, 1990.
96. Weiland AJ: Repetitive strain injuries and cumulative trauma disorders. Editorial. J Hand Surg 21A:337, 1996.
97. Wilbourn AJ: Thoracic outlet syndrome. Controversies in entrapment neuropathies: course D - 7th Annual Continuing Education Course. American Association of Electromyography and Electrodiagnosis, 1984, pp 28–38.
98. Wilbourn AJ: Thoracic outlet syndrome is overdiagnosed. Muscle Nerve 22:130–136, 1999.

ALAN L. COLLEDGE, MD
HUGH I. JOHNSON, MPA

S.P.I.C.E.—
A MODEL FOR REDUCING THE
INCIDENCE AND COSTS OF
OCCUPATIONALLY ENTITLED CLAIMS

From the Labor Commission, State
of Utah
Salt Lake City, Utah (ALC)
and
Utah Transit Authority
Salt Lake City, Utah (HIJ)

Reprint requests to:
Alan L. Colledge, MD
c/o Labor Commission, State of
Utah,
PO Box 146610
Salt Lake City, UT 84114-6610.

Despite remarkable advances in health care and increased emphasis on safety, ergonomics, and general employee health, the incidence and costs of workers' compensation and disability claims continue to increase. Today, the total cost of an average workers' compensation claim is estimated to be $13,182,[1] while the average cost of a lost-time (disability) claim can reach more than $20,000.[2] From 1985 to 1993, U.S. companies have seen their workers' compensation insurance premium almost double, with the cost now averaging 3.4% of the payroll.[3] Total costs for work-related injuries and illnesses in the U.S. have grown from $2.1 billion in 1960 to $171 billion dollars in 1997.[4] Of particular concern are common musculoskeletal injuries. Currently, 28% of all work-related injuries are soft-tissue musculoskeletal strains, accounting for approximately 40% of all lost-time injuries.[5]

Current literature indicates that the growth in disability from musculoskeletal discomfort is somewhat unique to modern western culture. Studies of third world countries show similar prevalence of discomfort (approximately 44%), but disability is virtually nonexistent.[6,7] Pain and discomfort is seen as an acceptable part of living. Interestingly, however, as western medicine becomes more prevalent in these countries, disability increases.[8] Historically, those who did the manual labor required in developing our modern society likely suffered musculoskeletal discomfort over the years, yet the record is mostly silent about disability. As with today's less-developed cultures, if they had pain and discomfort it appears they simply accepted it and made necessary adjustments in their lives. For all our good intentions, the remarkable interventions provided by modern medicine and businesses have not had a significantly positive impact on preventing or reducing disabilities.

Many individuals have a continual presence of discomfort in their lives. A recent study of 3000 randomly selected individuals showed that 14.4% of a general population experience carpal tunnel-like symptoms as a part of daily living.[9] Back pain shows a yearly prevalence in the U.S. population of 15–20%.[10] Among working-age people surveyed, 50% admit to back symptoms each year.[11,12] Most of these common ailments are benign, and recovery time is minimal. However, a small number recover much more slowly than expected and generate a considerably greater cost. A 1992 review of 106,961 workers' compensation low back injury cases found that approximately 86% of the costs were incurred by 10% of the injured workers.[13] A similar study of 21,338 work-related upper extremities injuries found that 25% of the claims account for 89% of the costs.[14] A State of Washington study found that the 5% of their compensation claims (accounting for 84% of the costs) are from individuals with nonverifiable muscle and back complaints.[15] Nationally, injured workers with skeletal fractures incur an average of 21 days off work, and those with amputations incur 18 lost days.[16] Yet patients with carpal tunnel syndrome complaints average 25 days away from work.[17] Similar studies have demonstrated that *compensated injuries have delayed recovery,*[18,19,20] *increased disability,*[21,22,23,24] *and decreased to return to work rates.*[25,26,27,28]

At any given time, up to 45% of currently employed workers could file work-related injury or disability claims, but most do not, choosing instead to carry out their job responsibilities, accepting some discomfort as part of living[29]. This **ability to tolerate discomfort** is determined by three primary elements: **(1)** the level of the biological stimulus (discomfort); **(2)** existing psychological distress; and **(3)** current personal social stress. Whenever one of these elements exceeds a personal toleration level, health care is sought (Fig. 1). Studies by Cameron found that those who sought assistance from health care providers reported more life stresses in relation to a sample of matched controls.[30,31] Zola found that individuals who sought health care did so because they could not stand their discomfort any longer.[32] A major international report from 15 centers in Asia, Africa, Europe, and the Americas reviewed 5,438 adults coming to health clinics with persistent pain during a period of 6 months or more during the prior year. Participants, who were interviewed and given psychological testing, were found to have rates of anxiety and/or depression four times higher than the normal population.[33] Of these, 48% had complaints of back pain, 42% joint pain, and 34% arm or leg pain. These results imply, as other studies have done, that psychological or social distress can be manifest as physical complaints that create a perceived need for professional health care.[34] In the workplace, psychosocial stress added to work activities can make even the normal discomfort levels associated with a particular job intolerable and result in a disability claim.[35] Often these complaints can have minimal or only coincidental relationship to the actual job tasks.

After becoming disability claimants these individuals can, by maintaining their symptoms, exert a level of control over their psychosocial stressors. With a medically acceptable physical diagnosis, the psychosocial concerns are legitimized, pride is maintained, and an unpleasant environment now becomes more socially acceptable.[36]

As these psychologically and socially stressed claimants enter the health care system, medical providers do as they are trained, i.e., mostly concentrate on relieving the physical complaints without addressing the social or psychological stressor. However, improvement is minimal since the individual cannot afford to improve physically—continued treatments validate the injury and solidify the role of a claimant and victim.[37] Treatments may become more varied and intense, but progress

Bio-Psycho-Social Balance

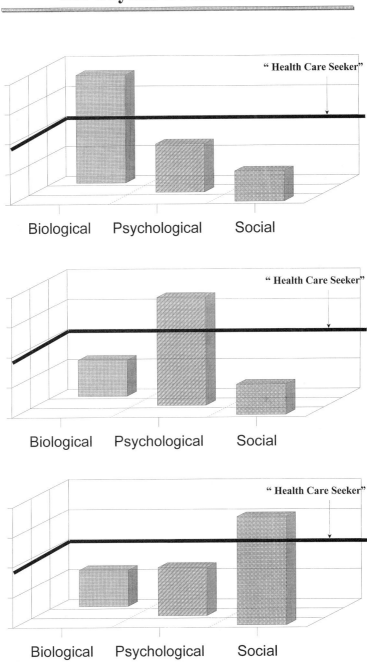

FIGURE 1.   Why people seek health care. The ability to tolerate discomfort is determined by the level of the biological stimulus (discomfort); existing psychological distress; and current personal social stress. Whenever one of these elements exceeds a personal toleration level, health care is sought.

is minimal, tolerance decreases, and symptoms worsen. As the desperate and anxious patient succumbs to more invasive and questionable procedures, disability is the natural result (Fig. 2).

This cascade may continue until some permanent disability occurs—a disability that is most likely the result of a discomfort level that could have been tolerable and nondisabling were it not for underlying social and/or psychological concerns. The medical and management system designated to help the injured individual instead creates more disability. A number of published reports have recognized such iatrogenic (system-induced) disability occurring within entitlement systems, and suggest the need for appropriate policy and management reforms.[38,39,40,41,42,43] More and more U.S. companies are offering higher levels of short- and long-term disability coverage to employees who find themselves unable to return to work as a result of both work and nonwork-related illnesses and injuries. With the federal government becoming more involved by passing legislation such as the Americans with Disabilities Act (ADA) and the Family Medical Leave Act (FMLA), the growth of disability seems poised for an unprecedented surge.

Nowhere is this more readily apparent than in **occupationally related back pain.** Occupational low back pain (LBP) is one of the most commonly encountered conditions in the industrial setting. Each year approximately 10 million employees in the U.S. suffer back pain that impairs their performance, and an estimated 1 million employees file workers' compensation claims.[44] Of the more than 11,500 complaints filed with the Equal Employment Opportunity Commission (EEOC) from July 1992 to June 1993, 18.5% have been for back impairments, making them the most common EEOC complaint, and monetary benefit awards have now reached $26.7 million.[45] In a survey of 12 states, the National Safety Council found that occupational back injuries account for 22% of workplace injuries/illnesses and 32% of workers' compensation costs.[46] Back pain is now the single most expensive category of industrial injuries, responsible for 31% of total industrial expenses, and is second only to

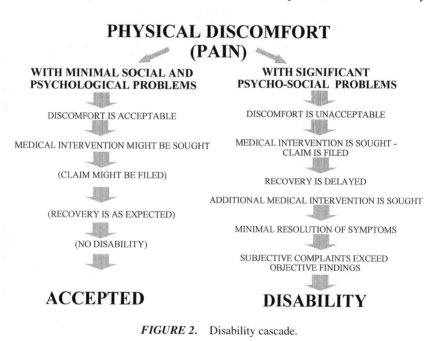

FIGURE 2.   Disability cascade.

the common cold as a reason for physician office visits in the United States.[47] Back pain results in a loss of 93 million to 250 million workdays per year and is the most common cause of disability in workers under the age of 45. Yet back discomfort appears to be part of living, with 28% of the adult population reporting current discomfort, and 50% of the population reporting back pain in the previous 6 months.[48,49]

Studies suggest medical or management tools that can affect this problem. However, as LaRocca stated, "This predicament is not the result of an inadequate fund of available information with which to address the matter. Instead the problem emanates from the lack of a comprehensive and unifying problem-solving strategy."[50] The quality of life for disabled individuals and their families, along with significant cost savings for business and industry, depend on identifying and instituting a dynamic, comprehensive system that decreases employee disability and maintains productivity. It is the authors' view that such a comprehensive, unifying, and dynamic model has been developed and validated over the years within **the military's "Forward Treatment" method** that prevents system-induced disability among battle casualties. Originally published in *The Journal of Occupational Rehabilitation* in 1993,[51] this model has been updated herein and expanded to include medical and management techniques demonstrated in literature and in practice to both prevent and manage injuries efficiently and fairly.

The model integrates medical and business management activities. Application of the model allows everyone involved with the disability management process to participate in reducing both incidence rates and costs.

S.P.I.C.E.

As today's medical providers and businesses struggle with increasing rates and costs from disability claims, it is important to note that during the past 150 years the militaries of the world have a developed a method of preventing delayed recovery and reducing system-induced losses.

Militaries discovered that when soldiers with relatively simple physical complaints were left to heal alone, or received inappropriate treatment for battle-related stress, some became permanently and totally disabled.[52] Placed under combat-induced conditions of anxiety and stress, the soldiers' protective psychological reserves eroded, and defense mechanisms began to form. Unchecked, these defenses transformed a relatively simple disorder, such as fatigue, into an "illness" that was both socially acceptable and serious. Further, once the "illness" was validated by the system, it released the soldier, either consciously or subconsciously, from the unpleasant emotional stress of his/her duties.[53] In response, the militaries evolved a successful treatment model, referred to as forward treatment, that prevents this system-induced disability.

During Israel's 1973 war with the Arabs, Israeli physicians noted that many soldiers had relatively minor physical impairments, yet behaved in a greatly disabled fashion. The best known medical care that could be given to these soldiers resulted in many of them becoming permanently disabled, with few returning to active duty[54] Treatment appeared to create iatrogenic or system-induced disability. Nine years later, during the Israeli war with Lebanon, Israel adopted the United States' Forward Treatment concept, and returned 60% of soldiers, with injuries similar to the 1973 casualties, to full duty within 72 hours.[55,56,57,58,59]

There are many similarities between military personnel and individuals involved in the disability/ workers' compensation environment:

1. Both groups are basically healthy. A certain degree of job-related intelligence has been tested for and is required, and those with pre-existing disabilities or serious illnesses have been screened out.[60]

2. Individuals are expected to function in terms of the needs of the team rather than the individual.
3. Both groups have legally mandated entitlement programs for "on-the-job" injuries.
4. The number and type of disability complaints are directly related to the intensity of psychosocial stressors to which the subjects are exposed[61]
5. Psychosocial stressors arise from factors other than the duty that the individual is exposed to. These factors may include personal performance, poor social support, team morale, duty satisfaction, personal belief in supervisors, and economic downturns.[62,63,64,65,66,67]

While certainly soldiers exposed to battle are highly stressed, many workers are likewise subjected to unprecedented daily personal stress that carries over into the workplace. Many employees feel that their lives are out of control as they deal with the difficulties of two-income families, care for elderly parents, experience reduced job security, and respond to increased expectations from employers.

These similarities suggest that 'Forward Treatment', validated on the battlefield, can provide an extremely useful model for the prevention and treatment of entitled individual's claims and costs.

This model, given the acronym **S.P.I.C.E.,** consists of five general components:

Simplicity—the concept that simple, benign conditions, treated in a complicated fashion, become complicated.

Proximity—the need to keep the worker associated with the workplace by building morale and support of employees

Immediacy—the need to deal with industrial claims in a timely manner.

Centrality—all parties involved with workers share a common philosophy and ultimate goal of returning the individual back to gainful employment as quickly as possible.

Expectancy—the concept that individuals often fulfill the expectations placed on them.

Simplicity

Simplicity comes from the military observation that ominous-sounding diagnostic terminology, complicated tests, and treatment for fairly minor problems (like battle fatigue) only served to strengthen the soldier's rationalization that he was indeed seriously ill.[68] Injured workers, like soldiers with stress, at times believe they are suffering from a serious ailment. For example, in one study 60% of back-pain patients believed or had been told that they had a "disc prolapse," although only 11% had any evidence of nerve root pain or dysfunction.[69] Another study of 140 patients with mechanical low back pain found that 67% were concerned with a serious illness causing their pain.[70] This contrasts with actual statistical experience that only 2% of persons with back pain may require surgery, and less than 1% have any underlying systemic illness.[71,72,73] Regardless of the cause of back pain, approximately 70% of affected people recover in 2–3 weeks, and 90% in 6 weeks.[74,75,76,77]

DIAGNOSTIC TERMINOLOGY

"Battle fatigue" has been closely tied with the history of warfare and has been given many names. During the American Civil War it was called "nostalgia"; during World War I, "shell shock"; during World War II, "war neurosis" and "combat exhaustion," and during the Korean War it was referred to as "combat fatigue." The more ominous sounding the "diagnosis," the worse the solder responded. Many times it appeared that the diagnosis given to stressed soldiers became a self-fulfilling prophecy, with the prognosis directly related to the initial label.[78]

Concerns about **diagnostic labeling** (which refers to the unintended, and usually adverse, consequences of simply assigning a diagnostic label to an anxious individual) have long been recognized. Researchers have shown that simply informing a person who feels that he or she has a 'disease' (such as asymptomatic hypertension) can cause an increase in 'sick behavior.'[79] For this reason, the military abandoned ominous-sounding labels such as shell-shock or war neurosis and replaced them with more benign names, such as 'battle fatigue' or 'combat reaction.'

The issue of assigning a diagnostic label has been identified in a review of 7,000 medical articles. This review showed that a pronounced lack of uniformity in diagnostic terminology is a major barrier to research and a key challenge to defining methods of treatment.[80] One study showed 20 current diagnostic terms ranging from the mundane "lumbar strain" to the exotic "Metameric Cellulotenoperiostomyalgic syndrome." In reality, only 10–20% of patients can be given a precise pathoanatomical diagnosis.[82]

Unjustified diagnoses must be replaced with **clear, nonthreatening terms** such as "simple strain." The physician should apply concepts of simplicity by: (a) providing an explanation of the most likely pain mechanisms; (b) reassuring the patient that serious disease is absent and; (c) providing information about the favorable prognosis of the natural history of the disorder. Business and disability claim managers should re-emphasize the simplicity of the diagnosis and discuss the likelihood of return to regular duty in the time frames given by the treating physician. Return-to-work programs should emphasize the physician's findings and allow light duty and other return-to-work activities that specifically follow the natural healing process of the injury.

TESTING

Sophisticated testing procedures can at times reinforce the severity of the "illness" to the injured worker. Physicians should limit the use of expensive diagnostic tests unless it is strongly suspected that the results of such tests would significantly change the course of treatment. For example, only one in every 2,500 cases of plain x-rays reveals a finding that is not suspected from a thorough history and physical examination.[83] Many imaging findings have nothing to do with the patient's current symptoms and are more likely the result of the natural aging process. A recent study of spinal MRIs in 98 asymptomatic subjects revealed that while 36% of the subjects had normal disks at all levels, 52% had at least one bulge at least one level, 27% had a protrusion, 1% had an extrusion, and 38% had an abnormality involving more than one intervertebral disk. Not surprisingly, physical findings increased with the age of the subject. The conclusion is that many asymptomatic people have disk bulges or protrusions, and the discovery of disk bulges or protrusions in people with back pain may often be merely coincidence.[84] In general, current image findings correlate poorly with back pain,[85,86,87,88,89,90,91,92,93,94,95] and are reported to be performed more frequently on workers' compensation patients than on comparative group health patients.[96] Because specific diagnoses are rare, and sophisticated testing procedures can have an adverse effect on the patient's illness behavior, adequate reassurance and education is often more effective in the long-term treatment of the compensated patient—and is no more time consuming.[97] Over-emphasizing the potential seriousness of a patient's symptoms can lead to the injured employee overreacting to them and can subsequently have a negative effect on recovery.[98]

Psychological Testing. Medical providers and managers dealing with claimants should be sensitive to the impact of somatic components and clinical inconsistencies on the long-term outcome of the case. However, extensive psychological tests are usually not needed during the first few weeks of treatment. Objectification can be measured by the process of establishing the medical history, performing a complete physical examination, the practitioner's effort assessment, and pain drawings[99,100,101] With this information, the practitioner can more readily quantify other subjective reports and findings of the examination.

Physicians must keep in mind the increasing volume of valid studies demonstrating the role of pain and illness behavior in certain patients. Do not immediately interpret behavioral signs of distress as physical disorders. The illness behavior component of a patient's disability can often be more important than the underlying presumed physical problem.[102]

TREATMENT

During World War II, the military used such exotic and complex-sounding treatments as 'narcosynthesis' and 'electroconvulsive therapy'.[103] The use of these treatment modalities often strengthened the soldier's rationalization that he was significantly physically or mentally ill.

Current treatments for musculoskeletal pain often fare no better than the exotic "cures" applied during World War II, and, like those cures, today's medical care has the potential to prolong disability by reinforcing illness behavior. Recent studies have shown that some medical providers are utilizing expensive, time-consuming treatment modalities, with little attention to efficacy.[104,105,106,107] As described previously, in third world countries where expensive diagnostic and treatment modalities are not available, there is little evidence of back disability being a problem.[108,109,110]

Note that of all procedures in routine medical practice, only about 10–20% has a basis in published scientific research.[111] This means that 80% of current treatment is somewhat subjective, explaining the significant practice variations that exist for treatment of some conditions throughout the U.S.[112,113,114,115,116] Outcomes, such as reporting those injured workers who are able to return to an occupational role, have been considered by some to be a "harsh" or "inappropriate" measure of success.[117] One study reported that 52% of injured workers undergoing spinal cord stimulation for pain obtained good to very good relief; however, less than 5% returned to any kind of work.[118] From the practical point of view, returning an injured/disabled worker back to productive employment is the ultimate measure of successful worker rehabilitation.

MEDICATION

In treating low back pain, strong narcotic medications may be contra-indicated, as they have been shown to delay recovery with significant complications and to be no more effective in pain reduction than milder analgesics such as aspirin (this is especially true if symptoms have been present for more than a few days).[119] In addition to reduced efficacy, narcotic medications have significant side effects, including tolerance, addiction, depression, and repression of endorphins. Tranquilizers are equally habit forming. When evaluating the effectiveness of muscle relaxants, the study results are mixed.[120,121] The most effective medications for reducing mechanical low back pain appear to be nonsteroidal anti-inflammatories (NSAIDs), such as ibuprofen and aspirin, which are relatively safe and inexpensive.[122,123,124]

Injections

A number of studies have looked at the use of injection procedures for the treatment of low back pain.[125,126,127,128,129,130,131] Infiltration of trigger points has not been shown to be particularly effective. Epidural injections of cortisone and local anesthetics have been the topic of a number of clinical studies, with variable results, and their use remains controversial.[132] Facet joint injections are also a common injection therapy. However, like trigger point injections, no significant studies are available to verify their effectiveness. Selective nerve root injections have, however, been proven effective in identifying the site of origin of the pain.

Bedrest

Over-emphasis on pain and discomfort alone and over-prescription of rest may indeed be a major factor of iatrogenic disability. The rationale for bed rest is the observation that intradiscal pressure is lowest in the lying position, and many patients actually feel better with bed rest. However, protracted bed rest leads to a catabolic state, with general malaise, bone demineralization, and loss of muscle strength.[133,134,135,136,137,138] There is also evidence that rest and inactivity actually inhibit healing and lead to increased psychological distress and depression, loss of work habit, and progressive loss of job opportunity.[139] Feeling better in the short term and getting better in the long term can often be two entirely different outcomes. *Return to normal activities should be the objective of all medical treatment and management efforts.*

Physical Medicine Modalities

Currently there is a marked increase in the utilization of physical medicine, now accounting for nearly 40% of the medical dollars billed in some states.[140] Yet traction, massage, electrical stimulation, ultrasound, thermal agents, acupuncture, manipulation, and diathermy have not been scientifically proven to heal tissues or facilitate healing.[141,142,143,144] Although these modalities may provide some measure of temporary symptom relief, there is little evidence that therapy modalities have long- term efficacy greater than a placebo and, unfortunately, modalities can create dependency and can distract patients from more responsible and effective treatment.[145]

Ergonomics

Although originally promising, prospective studies utilizing ergonomics and education have failed to demonstrate significant reduction in claims.[146] Ergonomic interventions apparently reach a point of diminishing returns. The 50-year quest to eliminate offending biomechanical stresses from the workplace has not had any positive impact on back pain or back pain claims in the workplace.[147]

Conditioning

The key to musculoskeletal symptom control is balancing mechanical stress against the more debilitating effect of inactivity on the protective musculature. Aerobic exercise, physical conditioning, and psychosocial support appear to be very beneficial for the worker with a soft tissue injury.[148,149,150,151,152] Recovery is inevitably dependent on conditioning of the protective and supportive musculature to compensate for any structural deficit caused by the injury. If strength is sufficient, a patient may return to full function—not because the back is cured, but because there is sufficient muscular compensation to tolerate the discomfort of activity.

SURGERY

Since the first article describing surgery for back pain appeared in 1934,[153] the number of spinal surgeries performed in the U.S. has increased exponentially. According to the National Hospital Discharge Survey, spinal fusion rates increased 200% from 1979 to 1987.[154] This increase in surgery appears to parallel an increase in related disability.[155] Too often, surgery is performed on patients who encourage it, expecting it to be a cure. Some patients, consciously or subconsciously, desire surgery to validate their disability, or even to assuage guilt.[156,157] The natural history of a herniated disc is to heal itself. Failure to operate very seldom produces serious adverse effects[158,159] Long-term outcomes demonstrate that nonoperative treatment of a disc herniation is often as effective as surgical intervention, and much more cost-effective.[160] In fact, Weber has demonstrated that surgery in the working-age group is a "luxury for speeding recovery when there are very strong preoperative indications."[161]

Application of Simplicity in treating and managing a disability claimant allows an approach to recovery that parallels the **natural history of the injury**. Intervention is provided at levels only sufficient for recovery. As the patient receives more efficacious treatment, there is a concomitant reduction in disability of patient and in costs for employers.

Proximity

"Proximity" deals with the need to create a work family both by developing worker morale and, when a claim occurs, by keeping the disabled individual as closely involved and associated with the workplace as possible.

Prior to 1917, the British army routinely removed 'battle-stressed' casualties from their duty stations, sending them home to England. It was assumed that returning the soldier to a more comfortable, stable environment would relieve the battle stress symptoms. Unfortunately, the reverse was found to be true. Many of those returned to England for battle stress became refractory to treatment.[162] After World War II, one-seventh of all military discharges were due to mental conditions. Of the 200,000 soldiers on England's pension list, one-fifth had a permanent diagnosis of "war neurosis".[163]

Later, in World War II, British and French physicians noted that soldiers with battle stress improved more rapidly when treated in permanent hospitals near the battlefront. The recovery rate was better still for those simply treated in casualty clearing stations near the front line. The most successful recovery was found in those **treated within the combat organization itself:** when encouragement, rest, persuasion, and suggestion (Simplicity) were offered close to battle lines (Proximity).[164]

The Israeli Defense Force (IDF) validated the concept of Proximity during the 1973 Arab-Israeli War and the 1982 war with Lebanon. In the 1973 conflict, all psychiatric casualties were evacuated to the rear of the battlefront. None of these casualties were returned to combat duty during the war, and many became chronically disabled.[165,166,167]

Sobered by the incidence of these psychiatric casualties, and the failure of the Israeli medical system to successfully rehabilitate any of them, the Israeli military adopted the doctrine of Forward Treatment, i.e., brief treatment (physical replenishment—water, food, sleep, and the opportunity to recount battle expe riences) near the front, with a rapid return to combat duty. To implement this new approach, the IDF deployed mental health specialists with each medical battalion, operating from 2 to 5 kilometers from the front. With this system in place, 60% of combat reaction cases were returned to combat duty within 72 hours.[168,169,170]

The second element of Proximity is the concept of **developing and maintaining morale.** The military found that in addition to battle intensity and battle stress, a variety of personal and unit factors influence whether an injured soldier performs well or becomes a psychiatric casualty: (1) confidence in one's own skills as a soldier; (2) belief in the legitimacy of the war; (3) trust in one's weapons; (4) confidence in one's comrades; and (5) trust in one's commander. In 1973, IDF soldiers from units with good leadership and unit cohesion, and who had stable personal and family lives, were less likely to become psychiatric casualties[171] and more likely to perform well and be decorated for heroism.[172,173] In 1982, good personal and unit morale also protected IDF soldiers from psychiatric breakdown.[174,175]

All those involved with managing entitlement claims must remember that working is one of the most potent modalities in preventing iatrogenic disability. Often the unhappy and disappointing aspects of a worker's home life can be mitigated at work. Work creates status and builds self-esteem. Work defines identity. It breeds self-reliance, provides personal security, and offers an opportunity for personal advancement. Through work we gain skills and develop personal efficacy.[176] Being away from work, especially as the result of a disability, encourages introspection and maladaptive behavior that can lead to increased illness behavior. Many workers, once injured, feel abandoned by their employers and coworkers. That feeling leads to erosion of the personal benefits of work. One major review of 8,500 injured workers in six states who were losing work time found that only 48% of employers had taken the trouble to call them during their recovery time, and only 33% of employers offered a return-to-work program.[177]

Proximity for the industrial worker is not limited to simply maintaining geographical closeness. Proximity includes all elements identified as generally **improving the physical, mental, and social work environment.** Perceptive employers agree with W. Edward Demming that the individual worker is the company's most important asset and that respect for individuals is paramount for business success.[178] Today, employees are under unprecedented stress due to marked increases in single parenting, divorce, teenage pregnancy, caring for grandchildren, and suicide. Consider the following demographic changes in the U.S. during the last 30 years:

- Illegitimate birth rates have increased more than 400%.[179]
- The percentage of families headed by a single parent has more than tripled.[180]
- The divorce rate has more than doubled.[181] Many project that about half of all new marriages will end in divorce.
- Teenage suicide has increased almost 300%.[182]
- Scholastic Aptitude Test scores among all students have dropped 73 points.[183]
- The number one health problem for U.S. women today is domestic violence. Four million women are beaten each year by their partners.[184]
- One-fourth of all adolescents contract a sexually transmitted disease before they graduate from high school.[185]

The challenge for employers is finding a means of developing a "work family" and assisting their employees in being able to come to work ready to give 100%, managing their life's stresses and fulfilling their individual goals and purposes in life. Indicators of the erosion of an individual's or employee's psychosocial reserves and an attendant potential for an injury claim can be indirectly measured by levels of tardiness, use of health insurance, quality of work, employee turnover, reduced productivity, accident and illness rates, property damage, grievances filed, and percentage of employees using employee assistance programs.

HUMAN RESOURCES

Personnel policies that are clear and evenly enforced can prevent undue employee frustration and help maintain a productive attitude among employees.[186,187] Occasionally, employees have an unrealistic idea about the financial benefits associated with being disabled. All employees should be educated about their rights as employees and what to expect, medically as well as financially, if a work-related accident occurs. A major review of injured workers found that 50% of injured workers had received no information from their employer about procedures to follow to get medical care.[188]

Qualified human resources staff should also provide channels for communication and dispute resolution. The majority of compensation-related litigation is arises from the frustration, ignorance, unrealistic expectations, and/or fear level of the injured workers.[189] Human resource policies that educate, accommodate return-to-work programs, and reduce anxiety in the worker also reduce litigation.[190,191]

In one study involving a geriatric hospital,[192] 46% of nursing aids initiated low back industrial claims, with an 82% recurrence rate. The hospital, in an effort to control these workers' compensation losses, implemented a program of back school training, with individual education on injury prevention and careful follow-up of reported injuries. A follow-up study revealed essentially no change in the injury and recurrence rates among their employees.

However, when this same hospital began a *personnel policy* of immediate contact following an injury and regular 10-day follow-up contacts, coupled with evaluation of retraining and early return-to-work possibilities, they found they were three times more effective in reducing time loss and recurrence rates for low back injuries. This hospital's experience clearly illustrates that making employees feel that they are valued and needed at the workplace can have a significant impact on the employer's bottom line.

In another study of 31,200 Boeing employees,[193] a strong correlation was found between the incidence of lost-time soft tissue injuries and a poor supervisor relationship. This was manifest through a poor appraisal rating performed within the 6 months preceding an injury. A similar study has been completed with urban transit operators.[194] These studies demonstrate that an employer's policies can often be more successful in returning employees to work in a timely manner and in reducing the number of claims, than medical personnel can be by treating subjective complaints.

SAFETY

A major review of injured workers found that only 44% had received special training or information on how to prevent injuries.[195] Companies using safety teams, videotaped safety meetings, incentives for worker participation, safety audits, safety management review of all accidents, placement of safety coordinators, and fatigue prevention programs have demonstrated a 30–90% reduction in claims.[196] Management commitment to safety should focus on identifying and reducing hazards, not just injuries.

DRUG TESTING PROGRAM

In 1990, the U.S. Navy found that 41% of sailors under the age of 25 tested positive for some drug use. Now, after 10 years of random drug testing, the rate has been cut to 2%.[197] Of 4,375 postal service employees nationwide that underwent pre-employment drug tests, 8.4% tested positive.[198,199] The group testing positive had 41% higher absenteeism, 1.5 times more involuntary turnover, and 1.7 times greater likelihood of quitting than the group that had negative drug tests. A major, 1-year study of 1,500 of the state of Louisiana's largest workers' compensation policyholders, implementing pre-employment, post incident, and random drug screening, demonstrated 50% reduction in workplace accidents and a cost savings of 22%.[200]

Unions

Many employers have found that rather than fight a union's involvement in their workplace, they can benefit from involving union officials in the development of safety and disability prevention programs. Unions should assist with lateral placement for injured employees, and establishment and enforcement of light duty or alternative duty programs, as mandated under the Americans with Disability Act.[201]

Wellness

The general health of an individual worker contributes to any incident that may occur and to the worker's response to that incident. A study of 1,652 firefighters tested several areas of general fitness including endurance, isometric strength, spine flexibility, blood pressure, and post exercise heart rate. Participants were divided into three groups—most fit, middle fitness, and least fit—based on the results of the testing. The subsequent worker's compensation back injuries and costs for these firefighters were then analyzed in relation to their prior fitness results. The frequency of subsequent injury for the least fit firefighters was ten times higher than that of the most fit group. The cost per claim for the least fit group was 13% higher than for the middle fit group. The most fit group had too few claims to make an accurate estimation of future costs per claim.[202]

Employers can contribute to a higher level of health and wellness by providing a worksite culture that encourages healthy lifestyles. Travelers Insurance Company, with 36,000 employees, introduced the Taking Care Program in 1986. Based on 4 years of experience, Travelers now reports an estimated return of approximately $3.40 for every dollar invested in health promotion.[203] Successful employee wellness programs feature: convenience, supportive corporate culture, management support, employee involvement in decision making, clear goals, and comprehensive, long-range planning.

Injury Response

When injuries do occur, the safety program should enforce the management's concern for the injured worker and the impact of the injury on other workers. Worksite injuries should be investigated, but not in an atmosphere of distrust. Investigations should focus on clarification of how the injury occurred, both to assist the injured worker and to take steps to prevent similar accidents from occurring in the future. This does not reduce the need to monitor all disability claims for potential fraud. However, an immediate positive response, while investigating facts of the claim, greatly increases trust and confidence in the system. With that trust established, fraud is more readily identified since the desire to "get back at the company" is greatly reduced.

Return To Work

Resumption of work has also been shown to be a significant part of the treatment for an injury or illness, even benefiting patients suffering from chronic pain.[204,205,206,207] Studies have shown that workers who return to their original employer are usually better off financially than workers who choose other options, such as alternative vocational rehabilitation plans that include retraining or new job placement.[208,209] Conversely, prolonged time away from work makes recovery and eventually returning to work progressively less likely. The longer an injured worker is kept from the worksite, the less likely it becomes that he or she will ever return to productive employment. [210,211] A recent study on the value of promptly offering modified duties reduced lost time by 30–50%. [212] Unfortunately, physicians, therapists, management, and labor all too often encourage disability by prolonging the injured worker's separation from the workplace. This is particularly true when the employer requires "100% recovery" prior to any work release. A 100% recovery policy may prove more costly to the employer than any other expense. Effective accomplishment of returning impaired individuals to work often requires the combined efforts of the individual, health care provider, and employer, to carefully evaluate the patient's ability and then, if necessary, consider efforts to provide reasonable accommodations. [213,214]

Applying the concepts of Proximity in the treatment of disability and occupational injury claims can significantly affect a company's profitability and employee morale, as well as reduce human suffering.

Immediacy

The need for immediate treatment was one of the first principles identified in dealing with soldiers suffering from combat reaction. Often, when there was a large influx of casualties, soldiers suffering from combat reaction were not treated immediately. Instead, attention was focused on more life-threatening injuries. Left to their own devices, these same soldiers were found to be more refractory to treatment when it was eventually offered, and more likely to need further rearward evacuation. The soldier's time away weakened his bonds with the unit and allowed him to solidify and rationalize the severity of his symptoms. In other words, a soldier near to his unit in space (proximity) and time (immediacy) can generally expect to return to it. This expectation decreases with distance, in space and or time.

A vivid illustration of the effectiveness of applying Immediacy was recounted in a *Wall Street Journal* article describing the aftermath of the 1985 crash at the Dallas/Fort Worth airport. [215] On August 2, 1985, windshear slammed a Delta L-1011 to the ground short of the runway. The accident severely injured many, and killed 137 people. In the immediate aftermath of the accident, Delta Airlines' management sought only for ways to comfort the bereaved. Within hours of the crash, the airline had dispatched employees to be with the family of every casualty. These Delta representatives provided clothing, financial aid, assistance in locating lost articles, and in general made themselves available to provide whatever was necessary at this most critical period in these families' lives.

As a result of the bonds created by this early intervention, many crash victims and their families found it difficult to sue Delta, whom they had come to see as a friend instead of an adversary. Of a possible 152 passenger claims in the crash, only 65 suits reportedly have been filed, and about 50 of these suits have been settled, most without litigation. This is impressive when compared with the 1982 Pan Am crash in New Orleans. In this incident Pan Am did not employ early bonding tactics, and at least 75% of the 146 passenger deaths resulted in litigation.

CRITICAL TIME PERIODS

Many clinical studies have validated the concept that timely treatment and return to work facilitates return to productivity. If, however, the absence from work is prolonged, permanent disability may be reinforced, and the chance to return to that job diminishes significantly. [216,217]

Within these studies of return-to-work parameters, several critical time periods have been identified. [218,219] All musculoskeletal soft tissue injuries should show some objective improvement within 2 weeks, regardless of the treatment imposed. Delay of expected time periods alerts the management team to potential recovery delays, triggering movement to a more aggressive treatment mode.[220] If pain persists beyond 3 months, treatment should expand to concentrate on psychosocial factors associated with pain that might be complicating the clinical problem.

Centrality

Centrality refers to the military's practice of making certain that all combat medical decisions, treatments, and evacuations are funneled through a central screening process. This ensures that only skilled personnel, trained in the Forward Treatment philosophy, are in contact with the solders at this critical period. This aspect of Centrality prevents the anxious soldiers from being exposed to confusing terminology, diagnostics, and treatments, thereby reducing iatrogenic disorders.

Too often in today's medical system a patient encounters a confusing maze of conflicting diagnoses and treatments. Specialists sometimes recommend tests that have already been performed, and often it is perceived that no one is directing care. With no one to take full responsibility for the direction of treatment, other members of the management team (the patient and employer) are confused as to what to expect and when to expect it.

To prevent this from occurring, health care providers must become more professionally coordinated, using the concepts of immediacy and expectancy in approaching the full spectrum of the patient's biological, psychological, and social needs. Often, at this point, like the soldier left to his own devices or subjected to inappropriate and uncoordinated care, the will or ability to work has been lost, disability is well established, and irretrievable harm has come to the patient and his or her family.

THE ATHLETIC MODEL

The team concept is not unique to the military. Athletic teams consistently rely on the collective energy and abilities of each member to attain success. It is well recognized that athletes recover from injuries very quickly. This efficient recovery is the result of a treatment model wherein common recovery goals are shared by a team, which includes the medical provider, coach, team members, and injured athlete. The result of this team approach is that an athlete, highly motivated and well supported, is able to return quickly to full function. If any supportive team element is missing or if the goal is not shared by all, return to activity can be delayed (Fig. 3). This model

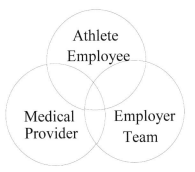

FIGURE 3. The team approach.

approaches treatment by sharing accountability equally among all involved entities with a return to productivity as the common goal (expectancy).

Just as with the injured athlete, the entitled (compensated) worker needs a structured, comprehensive approach to recovery. When the athletic model is applied, the worker becomes the "athlete," the employer takes the role of "coach," and fellow workers are the "team." **The success of this model depends on three components:** (1) motivation and physical capability of the injured worker (the athlete), (2) appropriate medical care, and (3) the desire of the employer (the coach) and coworkers (the fellow athletes) to have the injured worker return to work, manifested by the employer's willingness to support and accommodate the worker. Together, these components provide a structured and comprehensive approach to optimize recovery outcomes for the compensated worker. These include increased employee/employer communication; reduc tion in lost-time and associated, indirect costs; disability management; avoidance of litigation; and reduction of unnecessary medical costs. This approach ensures that all the patient's issues, including sociological and psychological concerns, are addressed, and obstacles to recovery are removed. Injured or disabled employees usually seek legal assistance because of misinterpretation and miscommunication. A multidisciplinary, centralized team approach could potentially avert such cases by resolving communication issues before they require litigation.[221]

EMPLOYEE MOTIVATION

Most compensated injuries are minor and heal uneventfully with little or no disability. However, in some injured workers, recovery can take longer than can be explained by physical symptoms alone, indicating the presence of nonbiological issues that serve to prolong the disability. A review of the medical literature demonstrates that compensation benefits alone can significantly affect motivation toward recovery.[222,223,224,225,226] The principal difference in recovery rates between compensated and noncompensated patients appears to lie in motivation—motivation of the injured employee, the employer, the insurance carrier, and government and medical providers. All parties involved in the recovery of a compensated patient are required to recognize the unique set of expectations, critical periods, and specific needs that must be met to attain return-to-work status.

Current research shows conclusively that in cases of delayed recovery, nonphysical factors often directly impact the injured employee's motivation.[227,228,229,230,231,232,233] These factors, often called "secondary gain issues," can prolong the disability. There might be a single factor or a combination of factors present, i.e. social, emotional, neurotic, economic, and even some times vindictive motives. Beneath this lies the original physical complaint that maintains the disability compensation payment.

Epidemiologic studies reveal distinct characteristics in the occupational and psychological profiles of people disabled by soft tissue injuries, particularly low back pain.[234,235,236,237,238,239,240,241,242,243,244] For example, job dissatisfaction, monotony, and stress are common characteristics. Persons facing these problems are more likely to suffer from depression, anxiety, hypochondriasis, and hysteria.

These nonbiological factors have an even greater impact on motivation when the entitled patient retains an attorney and becomes a legal claimant.[245,246] Once this happens, the patient is obligated to prove and preserve injury or illness. To improve physically jeopardizes the ability to prevail in a suit. Additionally, the worker's own credibility is placed at risk. Hence, the disability continues throughout the litigation process, even in the absence of any objective medical basis for the disability. Because legal counsel is usually sought only after a patient feels abandoned or "wronged" by the employer, personnel policies that prevent such adversarial relationships can have a significant financial impact on the company, as they may prevent costly litigation. Simple personnel policies can provide positive reinforcement for an injured worker, and also allow the employer to maintain control of an industrial claim.

TREATING THE TOTAL PATIENT — THE MEDICAL PROVIDER

Injured workers should be treated by clinicians whose treatment regimens have demonstrated the ability to effectively return the employee to work. Such clinicians must be sensitive not only to the biological pathology, but also to psychosocial issues that may limit motivation for return to work. In sports medicine, the provider must have an understanding of the game and knowledge of how the team interacts. The same principles apply in the occupational medicine arena. Clinicians who treat the injured worker should be comfortable with the type of work required for an injured worker to perform his/her job; this knowledge allows determination of the capability of the patient. These judgements carry heavy legal and ethical responsibilities, as fitness-for- duty decisions are often directly related to the individual's earning capacity and/or disability benefits. The status of current employment law indicates that any attempt to limit an individual's employability involves the need for a medical, legal, and ethical approach that protects not only the physician, individual, and employer, but the general public as well.[247] The clinician should also be well informed on workplace parameters such as the availability of modified duty.

EMPLOYER'S RESPONSIBILITY

Applying the concept of Centrality, employers have two main responsibilities: (1) prevent injuries from occurring, and (2) create a favorable return-to-work environment for the injured employee. To accomplish this the employer must understand and support the concept that timely work integration is critical to the rehabilitation of the injured employee. The injured employee should seldom be removed from work. Physicians should make medical determinations of physical capability, with administrative decisions regarding accommodations left to the employer.[248] Employers should evaluate medical restrictions given by the physician and make an administrative decision, in consultation with the medical provider, about when and in what capacity the injured worker may return to the worksite, whether in the same job or a modified position. Employers must be willing to accommodate early return-to-work during the rehabilitation phase, prior to the worker's full recovery.

RESIDUAL PHYSICAL CAPACITY

Many essential job functions require a significant amount of physical capability to perform. There is the eternal reality that we are mortal, and none of us will get off this planet alive. (Fig. 4)

We all arrive at points in our lives, irrespective of motivation, medical care, or employment concerns, when we physically cannot do what we would like nor what we once did. Just as injured athletes all reach a time when a change in careers is inevitable, so workers doing significant physical work will need to have serious discussion regarding accommodation of the labor-intensive essential functions of their work. Employers would do well to identify those jobs in which it is unlikely anyone could continue until retirement and develop plans to accommodate physical limits or, if necessary, shift aging workers to less physically demanding work.

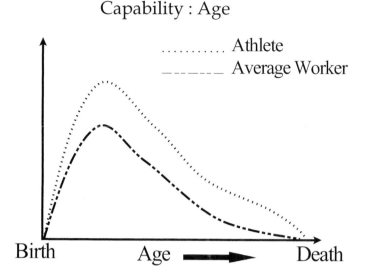

FIGURE 4. Every human being's capabilities decline with age, although the athlete's physical decline occurs at a higher level.

Expectancy

Expectancy, the final component of the SPICE model, reflects the fact that injured workers often fulfill the clinical and labeling expectations placed on them. Again, the military system provides a startling illustration of the role expectancy plays in the recovery of compensated individuals. Soldiers in World War I, who were diagnosed as suffering from shell shock indeed acted as if they had sustained a shock to the central nervous system. As recounted by Biley and others, "There were descriptions of cases with staring eyes, violent tremors, a look of terror, and blue, cold extremities. Some were deaf and some were [mute]; others were blind or paralyzed."[249]

When physicians realized that brain concussion was not the etiologic agent, as shell shock would imply, the term war neurosis was adopted.[250] This was hardly an improvement, as the general public associated neurosis with chronic and sometimes severe mental illness. The soldiers just as readily grasped this medical diagnosis as "proof" of their illness.[251]

Later, military medical personnel were instructed to label such casualties as "NYD (Nervous)" (for Not Yet Diagnosed-Nervous).[252] The term was obscure enough that it gave casualties little to cling to. This vague diagnostic label left the casualties open to the suggestion that they were just tired and a little nervous, and that with rest they would soon be fit for duty. Eventually, this disorder became referred to as simply exhaustion. In World War II, it was referred to as combat exhaustion. Finally, the term combat fatigue became preferable because it expressed more exactly the expectation desired, i.e., combat has fatigued the soldier, who requires only appropriate rest before quickly returning to full duties. The Israeli military has faced similar dilemmas in labeling combat fatigue.[253,254]

To fully understand why Expectancy plays such a vital role in human performance, it is necessary to recognize that belief or expectation can significantly affect the clinical outcomes[255] Some authors suggest that the pateint's expectations may influence outcomes more strongly than any clinical therapy.[256] Often referred to as the nonspecific effect of healing, or placebo, these effects have been reported to be strongest when the patient is anxious, the physician is perceived as having great expertise, the patient and physician believe the treatment is powerful, and the treatment is considered both impressive and expensive. The clinician's friendliness, warmth, interest, sympathy, prestige, empathy, positive attitude toward the patient, and positive attitude toward the treatment have all been found to significantly influence positively the outcomes.[257]

A review of treatments for angina pectoris originally believed efficacious, but later found to be ineffective or no better than placebo, have demonstrated 63–100% objective improvement,[258,259] far better than the usual 30% usually explained by placebo. Other studies have reproduced these findings.[260] A review of 2,504 diskectomies for lumbar disk disease that report negative surgical exploration found that 37% of the patients reported complete relief from sciatica and 43% complete relief from back pain,[261] results similar to those reporting positive disk findings at surgery.

Goals

Because there is little difference in effectiveness between assigned goals and self-set goals,[262,263] the physician is able to exert a healthy influence on patients' goals and expectations without prejudicing the clinical outcome.

Cathlove and Cohen utilized a "Directive Return to Work" approach in a multimodality rehabilitation program for workers' compensation patients.[264] Patients were divided into two groups—one directed in return to work, the other left to routine treatment with no specific return-to-work goals identified. In the directed group, patients were informed at program entry that they would need to resume work within 1–2 months. This return-to-work understanding was part of the initial treatment contract. The staff continually reinforced this concept by actively initiating return-to-work discussions and by guiding patients in setting work goals commensurate with their abilities. Sixty percent of patients in the directed group became gainfully employed. This is striking when compared to the nondirected group, in which only 25% returned to gainful employment. Nine months later, 90% of the directed patients who had resumed work were still working. In contrast, only 75% of the nondirected group who had returned to work remained employed.

The Physician's Role in Treatment and Patient Expectation

Often, patients unrealistically expect to be made completely well from a disorder or illness that is likely to leave residual symptoms. The lay press, family members, and other care providers often facilitate such unrealistic expectations. Left with symptoms and frustration with conventional health care, and receiving encouragement from peers and family, many desperate workers resort to aggressive surgeries or alternative health care therapies.[265] The goal is to provide the worker with realistic expectations of a disorder. This includes reviewing with the patient the risk and benefits of intervention as it compares to the natural history of the disorder and facilitating acceptance and independence. As with anyone left with a personal loss, these individuals will go through the five stages of grief outlined by Kubler Ross: denial, anger, bargaining, depression, and then, finally, acceptance.[266] (Fig. 5).

The physician must know how to recognize fixation at any level and assist the patient toward acceptance. One recent study matched treatment histories of 219 chronic pain patients under treatment at a multidisciplinary pain center and 185 former chronic pain patients who had not sought medical care for 1 year. Analysis demonstrated that the nonpatients had "learned to accept and live with their pain." The nonpatients demonstrated reduced levels of unrealistic thinking, less pain-related

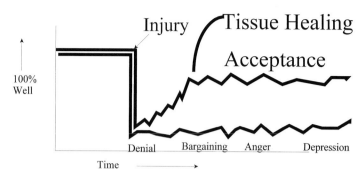

FIGURE 5. Physical and mental acceptance of injury.

distress, higher activity levels, and higher levels of internal orientation, and they required fewer medications. Researchers concluded "acceptance is a very legitimate goal for intervention."[267] Similar results have been demonstrated in other studies.[268] Physicians are mandated to be advocates of patients and of society, and in that role they should encourage ability, not disability. They should help patients retain a sense of purpose and self-worth that, for most, means a return to gainful employment.

CONCLUSION

Comprehensive problem-solving solutions are now mandatory to prevent the creation of costly disability. Medical providers, disability managers, and business managers must coordinate the redirection of treatment to the whole person, recognizing all the factors that influence successful return to work. Claude Bernard once wrote: "The greatest error in the advancement of medical science has been the search for a single cause for a single disease."[269] Or, as Aristotle said, "Treatment of the part should never be attempted without treatment of the whole. That is the error of our day, separation of the body from the soul."

The SPICE model, as outlined above, provides the much needed structure for comprehensive problem-solving strategies in preventing work-related claims and, when they occur, to deal with them in an efficient, fair, and timely manner, thereby preventing iatrogenic disability.

REFERENCES

1. National Safety Council, Accident Facts, 1998 Edition, Itasca, Il.
2. Attending Doctor's Handbook, Department of Labor and Industries, Revised June, 1999, pp 4. National council on compensation insurance.
3. US Department of Labor, Bureau of Labor Statistics
4. Leigh JP , Markowitz SB , Fahs M , Shin C , Landrigan PJ, Occupational injury and illness in the United States. Arch Intern Med 1997 Jul 28;157(14):1557–68
5. National Safety Council, Accident Facts, 1998 Edition, Itasca, Il.
6. Anderson RT: An orthopedic ethnography in rural Nepal. Medical Anthropology 8:46–59
7. Waddell G: The Back Pain Revolution, Edinburgh London New York Philadelphia Sydney Toronto. Churchhill Livingstone 1998, pp 4–5.
8. Waddell G: The Back Pain Revolution, Edinburgh London New York Philadelphia Sydney Toronto . Churchhill Livingstone 1998, p 5.
9. Atroshi I, Gummesson C, Johnsson R, Ornstein E, Ranstam J, Rosen I Department of Orthopedics, Hassleholm-Kristianstad Hospital, Sweden. JAMA 1999 Jul 14;282(2):153–8
10. Andersson GBJ. The epidemiology of spinal disorders. In: Frymoyer JW, editor. The adult spine: principles and practice.New York: Raven Press, Ltd.;1991. p.107–46.
11. Vällfors B. Acute, subacute and chronic low back pain: Clinical symptoms, absenteeism and working environment.Scand J Rehab Med Suppl 1985;11:1–98.

12. Sternbach RA. Survey of pain in the United States: The Nuprin pain report. Clin J Pain 1986;2(1):49–53.
13. Hashemi, L Length of disability and cost of workers' compensation low back pain claims, JOEM Vol 39, no 10, Oct 1997
14. Hashemi L , Webster BS , Clancy EA , Courtney Length of disability and cost of work-related musculoskeletal disorders of the upper extremity. J Occup Environ Med 1998 Mar;40(3):261–9
15. State of Washington Department of Labor and Industries, Attending Doctor's Handbook, 1996, p4.
16. US Dept of Labor Statistics, April 22, 1999
17. US Dept of Labor Statistics, April 22, 1999
18. Greenough CG, Fraser RD. The effect of compensation on recovery from low back injury. Spine 1989;14-.947–55.
19. Hunter SJ, Shaha S, Flint DF, etal. Predicting Return to work, A long term follow-up study of railroad workers after low back injuries. Spine 1998, Vol 23 No 21, pp 2319–2328.
20. Sander RA, Meyers JE. The relationship of disability to compensation status in railroad workers, Spine 1986;11:141–3
21. Guest GH, Drummond PD. Effect of compensation on emotional state and disability in chronic back pain. Pain 1992; 48:125–30.
22. Jamison RN, Matt DA, ParrisWCV. Effects of time, limited vs. unlimited compensation on pain behavior and treatment outcome in low back pain patients. J Psychosom Res 1988;32:277–83.
23. Leavitt F. The physical exertion factor in compensable work injuries; A hidden flaw in previous research. Spine 1992;17:307–10.
24. Milhous RL, Haugh LD, Frymoyer J'W, et al. Determinants of vocational disability in patients with low back pain. Arch Phys Med Rehabil 1989;70:589–93.
25. Fredrickson BE, Trief PM, Van Beveren P, Yuan HA, Baum G. Rehabilitation of the patients with chronic back pain: a search for outcome predictors. Spine 1988;3:351–3
26. Guck TP, Meilman PW, Skultery FK Dowd ET. Prediction of long-term outcome of multidisciplinary pain treatment. Ach of Phy Med and Rehabil 1986, 67 233–6.
27. Bednar JM, Baesher-Griffith P, Osterman AL Workers compensation. Effect of state law on treatment cost and work status. Clin Orthop 1998 Jun;(351):74–7
28. Milhous RL, Haugh LD, Frymoyer J'W, et al. Determinants of vocational disability in patients with low back pain. Arch Phys Med Rehabil 1989;70:589–93.
29. Biddle J , Roberts K , Rosenman KD , Welch EM What percentage of workers with work-related illnesses receive workers' compensation benefits? J Occup Environ Med 1998 Apr;40(4):325–31
30. Cameron L.: Symptom representations and affect as determinants of care seeking in a community-dwelling, adult sample population. Health Psychol. 12:171–179, 1993
31. Cameron, L., Leventhal, E. and Leventhal, H.: Symptom representations and affect as determinants of care seeking in a community-dwelling, adult sample population. Health Phychol. 12, 1993
32. Zola, I: Pathways to the doctor-from person to patient. Soc. Sci. Med. 7: 677–689, 1973
33. Gureje O, Von Korff M: JAMA July 8, 1998-Vol 280, No 2 147–151)
34. Ciccone DS et al.:Non-organic syptoms reporting in paients with chronic-non malignant pain. Pain, 68:329–41, 1996
35. Back Pain in the Workplace, Management of Disability in Nonspecific Conditions. Fordyce WE., IASP Press, Seattle Wa 1995.p.13.
36. G. Aronoff, 'Pain Need Not Be a Disability', American Back Society Annual Meeting pres. May 1990
37. Hadler NM , Arm pain in the workplace. A small area analysis, J Occup Med 1992 Feb;34(2):113–9
38. Cleland LG: "RSI": a model of social iatrogenesis. Med J. Aust. 1987:147:236–239
39. Stone WE: Repetitive strain injuries. Med J. Aust 1983:2:616–618
40. Browne CD, Nolan BM, Faithfull DK: Occupational repetition strain injuries: guidelines for diagnosis and management. Med J. Aust. 1987:140–329-332
41. Ferguson D. The new industrial epidemic. Med J. Aust. 1984:140:318–319
42. Ferguson D. "RSI": putting the epidemic to rest. Med J Aust. 1987:147:213–214
43. Hadler NM: Arm pain in the workplace. A small area analysis, J Occup Med, Feb 1992, 113–119.
44. Back Injuries: Costs. Causes. Cases & Prevention Washington DC: Bureau of National Affairs; 1988:80.
45. Equal Employment Opportunity Commission National Database as of 7-11-93, Office of Communication and Legislative Affairs. Washington, DC: EEOC.
46. Webster B. Snook S. The cost of compensable low back pain. J Occup Med. 1990;32:13–15.
47. Lemrow N Adams D Coffey R et al., The 50 most frequent diagnosis-related groups (DRGs), diagnosis, and procedures: statistics by hospital size and locations, DHHS Publication no. (PHS) 90–3465, Hospital Studies Program Research Note 13, Agency for Health Care Policy and Research, Public Health Services, Rockville, Md, Sept 1990.
48. Cassidy JD. Et al., The Saskatchewan Health and Back Pain Survey, Spine, 1998; 23(17):1860–6
49. Andersson GBJ. The epidemiology of spinal disorders. In: Frymoyer JW, editor. The adult spine: principles and practice.New York: Raven Press, Ltd.;1991. p.107–46.

50. LaRocca H: "Scientific approach to the assessment and management of activity-related spinal disorders"; Editorial. Spine Vol 12 No 7S 1987 European ed. S8
51. Colledge AL, SPICE—A Model for the Prevention Iatrogenic Low Back Pain Within the Current Workers? Compensation System, The Journal of Occupational Rehabilitation. Fall, 1993
52. Belenky, GL. Psychiatric casualties: the Israeli experience. Psychiatric Annals 17:8/Aug 1987:528.
53. Jones, FD, Hales, RE: Military Combat Psychiatry. Psychiatric Annuals, 17:8/Aug 87, p 525.
54. Belenky, GL. Psychiatric casualties: the Israeli experience. Psychiatric Annals, 17:8/August 1987:530.
55. Noy S, Levy R, Solomon Z: Mental health care in the Lebanon war. Isr J Med Sci 1984;20:360–365.
56. Belenky GL., Noy S. Solomon Z: Battle stress: The Israeli experience. Military Review 1985; 65:28–37.
57. Belenky GL, Now S, Solomon Z: Battle factors, morale, leadership, cohesion, combat effectiveness and psychiatric causalities, in Belenky GL (ed): Contemporary Studies in Combat Psychiatry. Westport, Ct, Greenwood Press, 1987.
58. Jones, FD, Hales, RE. Military combat psychiatry. Psychiatric Annuals, 17:8/Aug 87:525.
59. Bigot S, Nachemson AL. Work for all: For those with low back pain as well. Clin Orthop 179:77–85, 1983
60. Jones, FD, Hales, RE. Military combat psychiatry. Psychiatric Annuals, 17:8/Aug 87:525.
61. Bigos S, Nachemson AL. Work for all: For those with low back pain as well. Clin Orthop 179:77–85, 1983
62. Nachemson AL. Newest knowledge of low back pain. A critical look. Clin Orthop 1992;279:8–20.
63. Noy S: Stress and personality as factors in the causation of combat reaction, in Belenky GL (ed):Contemporary Studies in Combat Psychiatry. Westport, Ct, Greenwood Press, 1987.
64. Gal R: Courage under stress. In Breznitz S(ed):Stress in Israel. New York, Van Nostrand Reinhold Co, 1983.
65. Belenky GL., Noy S. Solomon Z: Battle stress: The Israeli experience. Military Review 1985; 65:28–37.
66. Belenky GL, Now S, Solomon Z: Battle factors, morale, leadership, cohesion, combat effectiveness and psychiatric causalities. In Belenky GL (ed): Contemporary Studies in Combat Psychiatry. Westport, Ct, Greenwood Press, 1987.
67. Gal R: Combat stress-An opportunity for heroism, in Belenky G L (ed): Contemporary Studies in Combat psychiatry. Westport, Ct, Greenwood Press, 1987.
68. Jones, FD, Hales, RE: Military combat psychiatry. Psychiatric Annuals, 17:8/Aug 87, p526.
69. Waddell G: An approach to backache. Br. J Hosp Med 28:187–219
70. Deyo RA, Diehl AK: Patient satisfaction with medical care for low back pain. Spine 11:28–30, 1986.
71. Deyo RA, Diehl AK: Patient satisfaction with medical care for low back pain. Spine 11:28–30, 1986.
72. Deyo RA, Diehl AK: Cancer as a cause of back pain: frequency and diagnostic strategies. Clin Res 35:738A, 1987.
73. Liang M, Komaroff AL: Roentgenograms in primary care patients with acute low back pain: a cost-effective analysis. Arch Intern Med 142:1108–1112, 1982.
74. Andersson GBJ, Svensson H-O, Oden A. The intensity of work recovery in low back pain. Spine. 1983:8:880–884.
75. Choler U. Larsson R. Nachemson A. et al. Back pain—attempt at a structured treatment program for patients with low back pain (in Swedish). SPRI Report 188, Social Planeringsoch Rational Isesingsinstitut Rapport, Stockholm, 1985:188.
76. Bergquist-Ullman M, Larsson U. Acute low back pain in industry. Acta Orthop Scand (Suppl). 1977–170:9–103.
77. Nachemson AL. The natural course of low baek pain. In White AA, Gordon SL (eds): Idiopathic Low Back Pain. St Louis, CV Mosby, 1982.
78. Jones, FD, Hales, RE: Military combat psychiatry. Psychiatric Annuals, 17:8/Aug 87, p526.
79. Haynes RB, Sackett DL, Taylor DW, et al: Increased absenteeism from work after detection and labeling of hypertensive patients. New Engl J Med 1978; 299:741,1978.
80. LeBlanc FE, et al: Scientific approach to the assessment and management of activity-related spinal disorders. 3. Dx of the problem. Spine Vol 12 No 7S 1987 European Ed. Supp 1, S16
81. Reference deleted.
82. Bigos SJ, Battie M. Overdiagnosis and over prescription of low back pain: acute care to prevent back disability. Clin Orthop. 1987,221:121–130,304.
83. Nachemson AF. The lumbar spine: an orthopedic challenge. Spine 1:59–71, 1976.
84. Jensen MC, Brant-Zawadzki M, Obuchowski N, et al. Magnetic Resonance Imaging of the Lumbar Spine in People without Back Pain NEJM July 14, 1994—Vol. 331, No. 2
85. Libson E, Bloom RA, Dinari G, Robin GC. Oblique lumbar spine radiographs: Importance in young patients. Radiology 1984 Apr;151(1):89–90.

86. Biering-Sorensen, F, Hansen FR, Schroll M, Runeborg O. The relation of spinal x-ray to low-back pain and physical activity among 60 year old men and women. Spine 1985 Jun;10(5):445–51.

87. Bigos, SJ, Hansson T, Castillo RN, Beecher PJ, Wortley MD. The value of preemployment roentgenographs for predicting acute back injury claims and chronic back disability. Clin Orthop Rel Pes, 1992 Oct, 283:124–9.

88. Fullenlove TM, Williams AJ. Comparative roentgen findings in symptomatic and asymptomatic backs. Radiology 1957;68:572–4.

89. LaRocca H, Macnab I. Value of pre-employment radiographic assessment of the lumbar spine. Indu Med 1970 Jun;39(6):253–8.

90. Hansson T, Bigos S, Beecher P, Wortley M. The lumbar lordosis in acute and chronic low back pain. Spine 1985 Mar;10(2):154–5.

91. Leboeuf C, Kimber D. White K. Prevalence of spondylolisthesis, transitional anomalies and low intercrestal line in a chiropractic patient population. J Manipulative Physiol Ther 1989 Jun;12(3):200–4.

92. Marora A, Schwartz A. Relation between the low back pain syndrome and x-ray findings. 1. Degenerative osteoarthritis. Scand J Rehab Med 1976;8:115–25.

93. Paajanen H, Erkintalo M, Dahlstrom S, Kuusela T, Svedstrom E, Kormano M, Disc degeneration and lumbar instability. Magnetic resonance examination of 16 patients. Acta Orthop Scand 1989 Aug;60(4):375–8.

94. Splithoff CA. Lumbosacral junction: Roentgenographic comparison of patients with and without backaches. JAMA 1953 Aug 22;152(17):1610–3.

95. Torgenson WR, Dotter WE. Comparative roentgenographic study of the asymptomatic and symptomatic lumbar spine. J Bone Joint Surg 1976 Sep;58(6):850–3.

96. Oleinick A, Gluck JV, Guire KE Diagnostic and management procedures for compensable back injuries without serious associated injuries. Modeling of the 1991 injury cohort from a major Michigan compensation insurer. Spine 1998 Jan 1;23(1):93–110

97. Deyo RA, Diehl AK: Patient satisfaction with medical care for low-back pain. Spine 11:28–30, 1986.

98. Nachemson AL. Newest knowledge of low back pain, a critical look. Cl Orthop and Rel Res. No 279 (June) 1992:16.

99. Nachemson AL, Bigos SJ: The low back, In Cruess RL, Rennie WRJ (eds): Adult Orthopaedics. New York, NY, Churchhill Livingstone, 1984:843–937.

100. Ransford AO, Cairns D, Mooney V: The pain drawing as an aid to the psychologic evaluation of patients with low back pain. Spine 1:127–134, 1976.

101. Waddell G, McCulloch JA, Kummel E, Venner RM: Non-organic physical signs in low back pain. Spine 5:117–125, 1980.

102. Nachemson AL. Newest knowledge of low back pain. A critical look. Clin Orthop 1992;279:8–20.

103. Jones FD, Hales RE: Military combat psychiatry: A historical review. Psychiatric Annals 17:8/August 1987: 526

104. Deyo RA. Conservative therapy for low back pain. JAMA 1983;250:1057–1062.

105. Koes BW, et al: The effectiveness of manual therapy, physiotherapy, and treatment by the general practitioner for nonspecific back and neck complaints—a randomized clinical trial. Spine Vol 17 No 1 1992.

106. Hadler NM: Diagnosis and treatment of backache. In: Medical management of the regional musculoskeletal disease. Orlando, Gurne & Stratton, 1984:3–52.

107. Spitzer WO, LeBlanc FE, Dupuis M, et al. Scientific approach to the assessment and management of activity-related spinal disorders. A monograph for clinicians. Report of the Quebec Task Force on Spine Disorders. Spine 1987;12:S1-S59.

108. Anderson RT:Orthopaedic ethnography in rural Nepal. Med Anthropol 8:46–59, 1984.

109. Waddell G: A new clinical model for the treatment of low back pain. 1987 Volvo Award in Clinical Sciences. Spine 12:632–644, 1987.

110. World Health Organization: Epidemiology of work-related diseases and accidents. Organization technical report series 777. Copenhaggen, Denmark, 1986.

111. Williamson JW, Braswell HR, Horn SD: Validity of medical staff judgments in establishing quality assurance priorities. Med Care 1979 Apr;17(4):331–46

112. Wennberg JE: Understanding geographic variations in health care delivery. NEJM 340 (1):52

113. Acute low back problems in adults: assessment and treatment. AGHCPR guidelines, No 14 Rockville, Maryland, Dec 1994.

114. Deyo RA, Cherkin D, Conrad D, Volinn E. Cost, controversy, crisis: Low back pain and the health of the public. Annu Rev Public Health1991;12:141–56

115. Keller RB, Soule DN, Wennberg JE, Hanley DF. Dealing with geographic variations in the use of hospitals: The experience of the Maine medical assessment foundation orthopaedic study group. J Bone Joint Surg 1990 Oct;72A(9):1286–93.

116. Volinn E, Mayer J, Diehr P, Van Koevering D, Connell FA, Loeser JD. Small area analysis of surgery for low-back pain. Spine 1992;17(5):575–81.
117. Fishbain DA, et al. The Prediction of Return to the Workplace After Multi disciplinary Pain Center Treatment. Clin J. Pain 9:3–15, 1993
118. Kupers RC, et al. Spinal cord stimulation in Belgium: Pain 56:211–216, 1994
119. Ohnmeiss P, Stith W. Gilbert P, Rashbaum R: Treatment of acute back pain in lumbar disc disease. Spine State of the Art Reviews 3:69, 1989.
120. Deyo RA: Conservative therapy for low back pain: distinguishing useful from useless therapy. JAMA 250:1057–1062, 1983.
121. Boyles WF, Glassman J, Soyka J: Management of acute musculoskeletal condition: thoracolumbar strain or sprain. a double blind evaluation comparing the efficacy of carispordal with diazepam. Todays Therapeutic Trends 1(1):1, 1983.
122. Deyo RA: Conservative therapy for low back pain: distinguishing useful from useless therapy. JAMA 250:1057–1062, 1983.
123. Nachemson A, with Spitzer WO, et al: Scientific approach to the assessment and management of activity related spinal disorders. A monograph for clinicians. Report of the Quebec task force on spinal disorders. Spine 12(7S) [Suppl.1];S1, 1987.
124. Cherkin DC: Medication use for low back pain in primary care. Spine 1998;23:607–614.
125. Nachemson AL: Low back pain, causes, diagnosis and treatment (in Swedish). The Swedish Council of Technology Assessment in Health Care. Stockholm, 1991.
126. Nachemson A, Spitzer WO, et al: Scientific approach to the assessment and management of activity related spinal disorders. A monograph for clinicians. Report of the Quebec task force on spinal disorders. Spine 12(7S) [Suppl. 1]:S1, 1987.
127. Jackson RP: The facet syndrome—Myth or reality? Clin. Orthop. 279:110, 1992
128. Marks R: Distribution of pain provided from lumbar facet joints and related structures during diagnostic spinal infiltration. Pain 39:37, 1989.
129. Nash TP: Facet joints—Intra-articular steroids or nerve block? The Pain Clinic 3:77, 1990.
130. Van Akkerveeken PF: Lateral stenosis of the lumbar spine. A new diagnostic test and its influence on management of patients with pain only. Rijksuniversiteit of Utrecht, The Netherlands, 1989. Thesis.
131. Jackson RP, Rae RJ, Montesano PX:Facet joint injection in low-back pain: A prospective statistical study. Spine 13(9), 1988.
132. Carette S, Leclaire R, Marcoux S, et al: Epidural corticosteroid injections for sciatica due to herniated nucleus pulposus. NEJM336 (23):1634
133. Deyo RA, Diehl AK, Rosenthal M: How many days of bedrest for acute low back pain? A randomized clinical trial. N Engl J Med 315:1064–1070, 1986.
134. Gilbert JR, Taylor DW, Hildebrand A, et al: Clinical trial of common treatments for low back pain in family practice, BR Med J 291:791–794, 1985
135. Hrudey WP: Overdiagnosis and overtreatment of low back pain: long term effects. J Occ Rehab Vol 1 No 4 1991:308.
136. Krolner B, Toft B: Vertebral bone loss: An unheeded side effect of therapeutic bedrest. Clin Science 64:537–540, 1983.
137. DeBusk RF: Cardiovascular responses to exercise in middle aged men after 10 days bedrest. Circulation 65:134–140, 1982.
138. Muller EA: Influence of training and of activity on muscle strength. Arch Phys Med Rehabil 51:449–462, 1970.
139. Bortz WM: The disuse syndrome. West J Med 141:691–694, 1984.
140. California Workers' Compensation Institute, October 16, 1997 97–19.
141. Cherkin DC, et al: A comparison of' physical therapy, chiropractic manipulation, and provision of an educational booklet for treatment of patients with low back pain. N Engl J Med 1998;339:1021–1029.
142. Hadler NM, Curtis P, Gillings DB, Stinnett S: A benefit of spinal manipulation as adjunctive therapy for acute low back pain: A stratified controlled trial. Spine 1987;1:703–706
143. Koes BW, et al: The effectiveness of manual therapy, physiotherapy, and treatment by the general practitioner for nonspecific back and neck complaints—A randomized clinical trial. Spine 17(1) 1992.
144. Acute low back problems in adults: Assessment and treatment. AGHCPR guidelines, No 14 Rockville, Maryland, Dec 1994.
145. Feine JS, Lund JP: An assessment of the efficacy of physical therapy and physical modalities for the control of chronic musculoskeletal pain. Pain 1997;71:5–23.
146. Daltroy LH: A controlled trial of an educational program to prevent low back injuries. N Engl J Med 1997; 37:322–8.
147. Hadler NM: Workers with disabling back pain. New Engl J of Med 1997;337:341–3.

148. Nutter P: Aerobic exercise in the treatment and prevention of low back pain. Spine 2(1), Sept 1987.
149. Bouchard C, et al: Exercise, fitness and health. A consensus of current knowledge. Chapt 45: Exercise, Fitness and back pain: Human Kinetics Books 533–540:1990.
150. Edwards BC, Zusman M, et al: A physical approach to the rehabilitation of patients disabled by chronic low back pain. Med J of Australia Vol 156 Feb 3 1992.
151. Estlander AM, et al: Effects and follow-up of a multimodal treatment program including intensive physical training for low back pain patients. Scand J Rehab Med 23:97–102, 1992.
152. Lindstrom I, et al: The effect of graded activity on patients with subacute low back pain: a randomized prospective clinical study with an operant-conditioning behavioral approach. Physical Therapy 72(4), April 1992.
153. Mixter WJ, Barr JS: Rupture of the intervertebral disc with involvement of the spinal canal. N Engl J Med 211:210, 1934.
154. The Back letter: A digest of current information and literature. Vol 7 No 6. 1992:1
155. Antonakes JA: Claims costs of back pain. Best's Review 9:36, 1981.
156. Goodwin PA: Prolonged disability for job-related injury. AFP Nov 1988:165.
157. Engel GL: Psychogenic pain and the pain-prone patient. Am J Med 1959;26:899–918.
158. Weber H: Lumbar disc herniation: A controlled prospective study with ten years of observation—1982 Volvo Award in Clinical Science. Spine Vol 8 No 2 1983.
159. Delauche-Cavallier MC, et al: Lumbar disc herniation—computed tomography scan changes after conservative treatment of nerve root compression. Spine Vol 17 No 8 1992.
160. Saal JA, Saal JS: Nonoperative treatment of herniated lumbar intervertebral disc with radiculopathy—An outcome study. Spine 14(4) 1989
161. Weber H: Lumbar disc herniation—A controlled, prospective study with ten years of observation. Spine 8:131–140,1983.
162. Jones FD, Hales RE: Military combat psychiatry: a historical review. Psych Annals 17:8/August 1987:525.
163. Jones FD, Hales RE: Military combat psychiatry: A historical review. Psych Annals 17:8/August 1987:526
164. Jones FD, Hales RE: Military combat psychiatry: A historical review. Psych Annals 17:8/August 1987:525.
165. Noy S, Levy R, Solomon Z: Mental health care in the Lebanon war. Isr J Med Sci 1984;20:360–365.
166. Belenky GL, Now S, Solomon Z: Battle stress: The Israeli experience. Military Review 1985; 65:28–37.
167. Belenky GL, Now S, Solomon Z: Battle factors, morale, leadership, cohesion, combat effectiveness and psychiatric causalities, in Belenky GL (ed): Contemporary Studies in Combat Psychiatry. Westport, Ct, Greenwood Press, 1987.
168. Noy S, Levy R, Solomon Z: Mental health care in the Lebanon war. Isr J Med Sci 1984;20:360–365.
169. Belenky GL., Noy S. Solomon Z: Battle stress: The Israeli experience. Military Review 1985; 65:28–37.
170. Belenky GL, Now S, Solomon Z: Battle factors, morale, leadership, cohesion, combat effectiveness and psychiatric causalities, in Belenky GL (ed): Contemporary Studies in Combat Psychiatry. Westport, Ct, Greenwood Press, 1987.
171. Noy S: Stress and personality as factors in the causation of combat reaction, in Belenky GL (ed):Contemporary Studies in Combat Psychiatry. Westport, Ct, Greenwood Press, 1987.
172. Gal R: Courage under stress. In Breznitz S(ed):Stress in Israel. New York, Van Nostrand Reinhold Co, 1983.
173. Gal R: Combat stress-An opportunity for heroism. In Belenky GL (ed): Contemporary Studies in Combat Psychiatry. Westport, CT, Greenwood Press, 1987.
174. Belenky GL., Noy S. Solomon Z: Battle stress: The Israeli experience. Military Review 1985; 65:28–37.
175. Belenky GL, Now S, Solomon Z: Battle factors, morale, leadership, cohesion, combat effectiveness and psychiatric causalities, in Belenky GL (ed): Contemporary Studies in Combat Psychiatry. Westport, Ct, Greenwood Press, 1987.
176. Panzarella, JP: The nature of work, job loss, and the diagnostic complexities of the psychologically injured worker. Psych Ann 1991:21:10–15
177. Out of site, but not out of mind, injured/ill workers and their experiences with workers' compensation system. A review of 8,592 injured workers in 6 states. Study commissioned by Intracorp.1996
178. Walton M: Thc Demming Management Method. New York, Putnam; 1986.
179. Monthly Vital Statistics Report. U.S. Department of Health and Human Services: National Center for Health Statistics, vol. 44, no. 11 (S), June 24, 1996.
180. U.S. Bureau of the Census, as published in the Statistical Abstracts of the U.S., October 1996, P. 99.

181. U.S. Bureau of the Census, Current Population Reports, pp. 23–180, and National Center for Health Statistics, Advance Data from Vital and Health Statistics, no. 194.
182. National Center for Health Statistics, Mortality Statistic Branch: Vital Statistics of the U.S.: 1975–1990, vol. 2.
183. U.S. Department of Education, The Condition of Education. The Office of Educational Research and Improvement, 1996.
184. E Byron Nahser and Susan E. Mehrtens, What's Really Going On? (Chicago: Corporantes, 1993), p. 12.
185. U.S. Bureau of the Census, Current Population Reports, pp. 23–180, and National Center for Health Statistics, Advance Data from Vital and Health Statistics, No. 194.
186. Fitzler SL, Berger RA: Attitudinal change: The Chelsea back program. Occup Health Saf 51:24–26, 1982.
187. Battie, MC: Minimizing the impact of back pain: Workplace strategies. Sem on Spine S, Vol 4 No 1 (March), 1992:pp 20–28.
188. Out of site, but not our of mind, injured/ill workers and their experiences with workers' compensation system, Study commissioned by Intracorp.1996
189. California Workers' Compensation Institute Report To the Governor and Legislature, July 1985
190. Out of site, but not our of mind, injured/ill workers and their experiences with workers' compensation system, A review of 8,592 injured workers in 6 states. Study commissioned by Intracorp.1996
191. California Workers' Compensation Institute Report To the Governor and Legislature, July 1985
192. Wood DJ: Design and evaluation of a back injury prevention program within a geriatric hospital. Spine Vol 12 No 2 1987.
193. Bigos S, Nachemson AL: Work for all: For those with low back pain as well. Clin Orthop 179, 1983.
194. Krause N: Psychosocial Job Factors, Physcial Workload, and Incidence of Work Related Spinal Injury: A 5 yr Prospective Study of Urban Transit Operators. Spine 23(23):2507–2516.
195. Out of site, but not our of mind, injured/ill workers and their experiences with workers' compensation system, A review of 8,592 injured workers in 6 states. Study commissioned by Intracorp.1996
196. Workers' Compensation Monitor, July 1998 p10
197. Burt, M. R., M. M. Biegel, Y. Carnes, and E. C. F-arley. Worldwide Highlights From the Worldwide Survey of Non-Medical Drug Use and Alcohol Use Among Military Personnel Bethesda, Md.: Burt Associates; 1980.
198. Normand, J. Relationship between drug test results and job performance indicators. Presented at the 97th American Psychological Association meeting, New Orleans, La.; 1989.
199. Zwerling, C., J. Ryan, and E. J. Orav. The efficacy of preemployment drug screening for marijuana and cocaine in predicting employment outcome. JAMA 1990;264:2,639–2,643.
200. Creating a Drug Free Workplace,: How to Design and Implement an Effective program Louisiana Workers' Compensation Crop, 800-756-7123
201. Americans with Disabilities Act 42 USC § 12101 (1991).
202. Lee D. Cady, MD, et al.: Strength and Fitness and Subsequent Back injuries in Firefighters. Journal of Occupational Medicine ? Vol 21, No. 4/April 1979
203. Lynch WD, Golaszewski TJ, Clearie AF, Snow D, Vickery DM, *Impact of a facility-based corporate fitness program on the number of absences from work due to illness.* J Occup Med 1990 Jan;32(1):9–12
204. Dent GL.Curing the disabling effects of employee injury. Risk Manage. 1985; January:30.
205. Derebery VJ, Tullis WH. Delayed recovery in the patient with a work compensable injury. J Occup Med 1983;25:829–835.
206. Nachemson AL. Work for all. Clin Orthop. 1983;179:77.
207. Mayer TG, Gatchel RJ, Kishono N. et al. Objective assessment of spine function following industrial injury: a prospective study with comparison group and one year follow up. Spine. 1985;10:483–493.
208. Gice J. Tomokins K. Cutting costs with return to work programs. Risk Manage. 1988;35:62–65.
209. Taylor T. Working around workers' injuries. Nation's Business. 1988;76:39–40.
210. Dworkin RH, Handlin DS, Richlin DM, Brand L Vannucci C Unraveling the effects of compensation, litigation, and employment on treatment response in chronic pain. Pain. 1985;23:49–59.
211. Stung JP. The chronic disability syndrome. In: Aronoff GM, ed. Evaluation and Treatment of Chronic Pain. Baltimore, MD: Urban & Schwarzenberg; 1985.
212. Yassi A, Tate R, Cooper JE, Snow C, Vallentyne S, Khokhar JB Early intervention for back-injured nurses at a large Canadian tertiary care hospital: an evaluation of the effectiveness and cost benefits of a two-year pilot project.Occup Med (Lond) 1995 Aug;45(4):209–14
213. Americans with Disabilities Act 42 USC § 12101 (1991).
214. Ryden LA, Molgaard CA, Bobbitt SL Benefits of a back care and light duty health promotion program in a hospital setting. J Community Health 1988 Winter;13(4):222–30
215. Bean E: Damage control- after 137 people died in its Texas jet crash, Delta helped families. Wall Street Journal Nov 7 1988.

216. Dworkin RH, Handlin DS, Richlin DM, Brand L Vannucci C Unraveling the effects of compensation, litigation, and employment on treatment response in chronic pain. Pain. 1985;23:49–59.
217. Stung JP. The chronic disability syndrome. In: Aronoff GM, ed. Evaluation and Treatment of Chronic Pain. Baltimore, MD: Urban & Schwarzenberg; 1985.
218. Nachemson A, et al: Management guidelines. Spine Vol 12 No 7s September, 1987 European ed Supp 1.
219. Nachemson A: Work for all—for those with low back pain as well. Cl Orthop and Related Research No 179 Oct 1983, 78–80.
220. Acute low back problems in adults: assessment and treatment. AGHCPR guidelines, No 14 Rockville, Maryland, Dec 1994.
221. Litigation and workers' compensation: a report to industry, Report to the governor and California legislature, July 1979
222. Symptoms may return after carpal tunnel surgery, JAMA, April 17, 91, Vol 265, No 15.
223. Butler RJ. Worral JD: Worker injury compensation the duration of non-work spells. Econ J 95:714–724, 1985.
224. Worral JD. Appel D: The impact of workers' compensation benefits on low back claims. In Hadler NM (ed): Clinical Concepts in Regional Musculoskeletal Illness. Orlando, Grune and Stratton. 1987:281–297.
225. Worral JD. Butler RJ: Benefits and claim duration. In Worral JD, Appel D (eds): Workers' Compensation Benefits: Adequacy, Equity and Efficiency: Ithaca, ILR Press. 1985:57–70.
226. Sander RA, Meyers JE: The relationship of disability to compensation status in railroad workers. Spine 11:141–143, 1984
227. Hunter, S Predicting Return to Work, A long-term follow-up study of Railroad workers After Low Back Injuries, Spine Vol 32, No 21, pp 2319–2328. 1998
228. Bigos SJ, Andary MT: The practitioner's guide to the industrial back problem: part I. Helping the patient with the symptoms and pathology. Sem in Spine S. Vol 4 No 1 (March):42–54; 1992.
229. Brodsky CM: Psychological factors contributing to somatoform disease attributed to the workplace. the case of intoxication. J Occup Med 1983;25:459–64.
230. Hirschfeld AH, Behan RC: The accident process. I. etiological considerations of industrial injuries. JAMA 1963; 186:193–9.
231. Florence DLO, Miller TC: Functional overlay in work-related injury. A system for differentiating conscious from subconscious motivation of persisting symptoms. Postgrad Med 1985; 77(8):97–100, 104, 108.
232. Frymoyer JW, Cats-Baril W: Predictors of low back pain disability. Cl Ortho and Related Res: No 221 August 1987;89–96.
233. Roles of Fatigue, Tension in recurrent low back pain. Family Practice News April 1–14, 1988:pp. 16
234. Mangnusson, M. Granqvist M, et al. The loads on the lumbar spine during work at an assembly line. The risks for fatigue injuries of vertebral bodies. Spine Vol 15 No 8:774; 1990.
235. Magora A: Investigation of the relation between low back pain and occupation. V. Psychological aspects. Scand J Rehabil Med 5:191–196, 1973.
236. Romano JM, Turner JA: Chronic pain and depression: does the evidence support a relationship? Psych. Bull. 97:18, 1985.
237. Bigos SJ Battie MC, Fisher LD, Fordyce WE, Hansson TH, Nachemson AL, Spengler DM: A prospective study of work perceptions and psychosocial factors affecting the report of back injury. Spine 16(1):(in press), 1990.
238. Westin CG: Low back sick-listing: a nosological and medical insurance investigation. Scand J Soc Med (Supp 7): 1–116, 1973.
239. Craufurd DIO, Creed F, Jayson MIV: Life events and psychological disturbances in patients with low back pain. Spine Vol 15 No 6 1990.
240. Gallagher RM, et al: Determinants of return-to-work among low back pain patients. Pain 39(1989) 55–67.
241. Weinstein MR: The concept of the disability process. Psychosomatics 1978:19:94–7.
242. Vallfors B: Acute, subacute and chronic low back pain: clinical symptoms, absenteeism and working environment. Scand J. Rehabil Med [Supp] 1985;11:1–98.
243. Anderson GJB, Svensson HO, Oden A: The intensity of work recovery in low back pain. Spine 19843;8:880–4
244. Frymoyer JW, Rosen JC, Clements J, Pope MH: Psychologic factors in low back pain disability. Clin Orthop 1985; 195:178–84.
245. Litigation and workers' compensation: a report to industry, Report to the governor and California legislature, July 1979
246. Hunter SJ, Shaha S, Flint DF, etal. Predicting Return to work, A long term follow-up study of railroad workers after low back injuries. Spine 1998, Vol 23 No 21, pp 2319–2328
247. Americans with Disabilities Act 42 USC, §12101 (1991).

248. Americans with Disabilities Act 42 USC § 12101 (1991).

249. Bailey P, Williams FE, Komora PO: The medical department of the United States Army in the World War, Volume X, Neuropsychiatry. US Government Printing Office, 1929.

250. Farrar CB: War and neurosis. American Journal of Insanity 1917; 73:12.

251. Jones FD, Hales RE: Military combat psychiatry: a historical review. Psych Annals 17:8/Aug 1987;526.

252. Jones FD, Hales RE: Military combat psychiatry: a historical review. Psych Annals 17:8/Aug 1987;526

253. Belenky GL: Psychiatric casualties: the Israeli experience. Psych Annals 17:8/Aug 1987

254. Jones FD, Hales RE: Military combat psychiatry: a historical review. Psych Annals 17:8/Aug 1987;526

255. Hall H, Iceton JA: Back school: An overview with specific reference to the Canadian back education units. Clin Orthop 179:10, 1983.

256. Repko GR, Cooper R: A study of the average workers' compensation case. J Clin Psych 39:287–295, 1983.

257. Turner JA , Deyo RA , Loeser JD , Von Korff M , Fordyce WE The importance of placebo effects in pain treatment and research JAMA 1994 May 25;271(20):1609–14.

258. Diamond EG, Comparison of internal mammary ligation and sham operation for angina pectoris. Am J Caridol 1960;5:483–486

259. Cobb, LA An evaluation of internal mammary artery ligation by a double blind technique, N Engl j Med. 1959;260:1115–1118

260. Goodman P. Response of patients with myofacial pain dysfunction syndrome to mock equilibration. J Am Dent Assoc, 1976;93:755–758.

261. Spangfort EV. The lumbar disc herniation: A computer aided analysis of 2504 operation. Acta Othoop Scand. 1972:142(suppl):1–95

262. Ashworth DN: An experimental study of the effects of three participative goal setting strategies on perception of goal difficulty, goal acceptance, satisfaction and task performance. Diss Abstr Int 1980;40(12):6344.

263. Alexy B: Goal setting and health risk reduction. Nurs Res 1985;34(5):283–8.

264. Catchlove R. Cohen K: Effects of a directive return to work approach in the treatment of workmans' compensation patients with chronic pain. Pain 14:181–191.,1982.

265. Astin JA,Why patients use alternative medicine: results of a national JAMA 1998 May 20;279(19):1548–53

266. Noyes R Jr , Clancy J The dying role: its relevance to improved patient care. Psychiatry 1977 Feb;40(1):41–7

267. Reitsma B , Meijler WJ, Pain and patienthood. Clin J Pain 1997 Mar;13(1):9–21

268. Lorig KR , Mazonson PD , Holman HR Evidence suggesting that health education for self-management in patients with chronic arthritis has sustained health benefits while reducing health care costs. Arthritis Rheum 1993 Apr;36(4):439–46

269. Bernard C: An introduction to the study of experimental medicine, Green HC (Trans), New York, Dover, 1957

ALAN L. COLLEDGE, MD
RICHARD E. JOHNS, JR, MD, MSPH

UNIFIED FITNESS REPORT FOR THE WORKPLACE

From the Labor Commission, State
Of Utah (AC)
Salt Lake City, Utah
and
Alliant Techsystems (RJ)
Magna, Utah

Reprint request to:
Alan L. Colledge, MD
c/o Labor Commission, State of
Utah
PO Box 146610
Salt Lake City, UT 84114-6610.

Fitness statements often are required of physicians by patients, employers, governmental agencies, and insurance providers to determine if a patient is fit for duty. Physicians making these ability statements are legally obligated to carefully justify them, as they determine placement or exclusion of individuals from the workplace. The Americans with Disabilities Act (ADA) mandates that medical providers use justifiable criteria and rational thought when determining the capability and risk of an individual. This chapter reviews the legal requirements of the ADA for employers and physicians and presents a uniform methodology that both could use to determine the performance capability of an individual with a temporary or permanent impairment or disability.

It is increasingly common for physicians, irrespective of medical specialty, to be asked to determine an individual's physical, mental, or social abilities, for either temporary or permanent work. Those requesting this information include government agencies (social security, state welfare, employment security, labor commissions, vocational rehabilitation, driver's license divisions) employers, insurance payers (workers' compensation, short- and long-term disability, Family Medical Leave Act qualifications), and loan deferment officers. Each requests the same basic information with a plethora of significantly different and time-consuming forms. The interest in medically objectifiable and legally defensible abilities and risk statements is increasing, as most agencies requesting this information are experiencing significant increases in disability applications and costs. For example, from 1970 the Federal Government has seen individuals awarded Social Security Disability

Insurance (SSDI) and Supplemental Security Income (SSI) double. At the end of 1992, approximately 8.8 million people were receiving SSDI and/or SSI benefits for a total cost of $52 billion.[1] Likewise, U.S. employers have seen their costs for work-related injuries and associated disabilities increase from $2.1 billion in 1960 to an annual estimated total cost of $171 billion a year.[2] Currently, the average cost of a lost-time work-related injury is more than $20,000.[3] It is now estimated that at least 43 million Americans are disabled in some way. However, 60% of those not working have indicated that they would like to work if the opportunity were made available,[4] and 25% of disabled individuals have reported some form of current job discrimination.[5]

Medically determined physical-ability-and-risk statements are the first step toward the final administrative disposition as to whether a person is deemed fit or unfit for duty (Fig. 1). These ability decisions carry heavy legal and ethical responsibilities, because fitness-for-duty decisions often are directly related to the individual's earning capacity and/or disability benefits. Current employment law indicates that any attempt to limit an individual's employability involves the need for a medical, legal, and ethical approach that protects not only the physician, individual, and employer, but the general public as well.[6] In the past, there was minimal research available predicting who would become disabled, so physical-ability-and-risk statements were made intuitively by medical providers.[7,8,9,10]

Generally, treating physicians cannot be sued for their opinions concerning an individual's ability to work unless a physician's statement is proved false and was made with recklessness. However, physicians can be sued for negligent interference with the worker's contractual relationship.[11] Therefore, all who are involved with physical ability decisions must realize that physicians determine *ability,* not disability. Generally, it is not the physician's responsibility to tell the employer whether the employee can do his or her job, determine the essential functions of the job, devise accommodations for the individual, or determine the reasonableness of any accommodation proposed by the employer. Employability, accommodation, and disability decisions are administrative.

In making physical ability statements, physicians should be cognizant that returning individuals to gainful employment is one of the most potent therapeutic and rehabilitative modalities available. Work promotes independence and is essential to a person's self-respect and quality of life.[12] Resumption of work also has been shown to be a significant part of the treatment for an injury or illness, even benefiting pa-

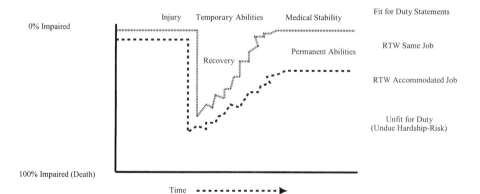

FIGURE 1.   Recovery graph.

tients suffering from chronic pain.[13,14,15,16] Conversely, prolonged time away from work makes recovery and eventually returning to work progressively less likely.[17,18] American industry has come to appreciate W. Edwards Demming's philosophy that the "individual worker is the company's most important asset, and respect for individuals is paramount for business success."[19] Studies have shown that workers who return to their original employer are usually better off financially than workers who choose other options, such as alternative vocational rehabilitation plans that include retraining or new job placement.[20,21] Many companies now sponsor modified work programs before full duty is assumed. Effective accomplishment of returning impaired individuals to work often requires the combined efforts of the individual, healthcare provider, and employer, to carefully evaluate the patient's ability and then, if necessary, consider efforts to provide reasonable accommodations.[22]

FITNESS FOR DUTY UNDER ADA

The ADA is a civil rights law that prohibits discrimination in public and private employment, governmental services, public accommodations, public transportation, and telecommunication. Its prohibitions apply to employers with 15 or more employees and to state and local governments and public services of any size. The ADA specifically protects all individuals with a physical or mental impairment that substantially limits one or more of the major life activities; with a record of such impairment; and regarded as having such an impairment. This law protects injured individuals, those who acquire various diseases, and those who have lifetime disabilities and may have never worked. The ADA also is designed to assist employers in managing the effects of individuals' disabilities and places very specific requirements on employees, employers, and their medical advisors to determine the conditions under which individuals can work.[23]

Under the ADA, it is no longer sufficient for a physician simply to determine if a person is disabled. Capability must first be ascertained before other administrative issues such as "reasonable accommodation," "undue hardship," or "direct threat"[24] can be addressed. Failure to comply with the ADA may result in costly litigation. Originally it was thought the ADA would primarily prevent discrimination in the hiring process; however, the enforcing agency, the Equal Employment Opportunity Commission, reports that 52% of cited violations relate to wrongful discharge of an employee, 27% to failure to provide reasonable accommodation, and only 10% to hiring practices.[25] Physicians can unwittingly provide a trigger for ADA coverage by recommending work restrictions focused on what an employee is unable to do and not relating the restrictions to the particular specific functions of the job at issue.[26]

DIRECT THREAT

In order for an employer to determine if an individual is unfit for his or her current job, or whether a job offer should be withdrawn based on a physician's recommendations, it must be shown that the individual poses a high probability of causing substantial harm to self or others, and that the risk of substantial harm cannot be eliminated or reduced below the direct threat level by reasonable accommodation.[27] This is a very stringent standard that most employers and physicians rarely are able to meet when attempting to screen for potential future injury, in that medical science rarely produces data that demonstrates a *"high probability"* that something bad will happen. Probability is a term that refers to the likelihood or chance that an injury or illness was caused or aggravated by a particular factor. "Possibility" sometimes is used to imply a likelihood of less than 50%; "probability" sometimes is used to imply a likelihood of greater than 50%.[28] Moreover, such claims cannot be speculative or based on potential future risk. Only the current abilities of the individual to perform essential job functions safely can be assessed.

EMPLOYER RESPONSIBILITIES

Given appropriate medical abilities information, an employer's administrative responsibility is to determine whether reasonable accommodations can be made. If the employer feels that accommodations represent an "undue hardship" for the company, or that the employee is considered a "threat to self or others," an employability decision by management of the individual being unfit for duty is made. Such action requires appropriate legal review and significant documentation. The decision may depend on a number of variables, including the size of the employer's organization, their resources available, and the nature of the operation.[29,30] Whether a particular accommodation will impose an undue hardship must be determined on a case-by-case basis. [31,32] An accommodation that poses an undue hardship for one employer at a particular time may not pose an undue hardship for another employer or the same employer at another time. Factors to be considered in determining whether an accommodation would create an undue hardship on a particular business are reviewed in greater detail in the ADA and Technical Assistance Manual.[33]

UNIFIED FITNESS MEDICAL REPORT

A number of contributing variables, including the history and physical examination, medical testing results, diagnosis, functional capacity evaluations, compliance with treatment guidelines, and medical outcome studies, may need to be considered in arriving at a fitness-for-duty statement (Fig. 2). Comprehensive functional abilities can be determined via 21 different categories from which individual health concerns may arise (Table 1).

To facilitate this complicated process, the Utah Medical Association (UMA) has developed a novel interdisciplinary approach, referred to as The Unified Fitness Report (UFR).[34] These guidelines were developed in a similar format as the Utah Driver License Division's health form and by a consensus of 28 specialists of the UMA, with consideration of the ethical and legal liabilities that physicians, ergonomists, attorneys, business managers, and supervisors experience in balancing the patient's and societal interests as required under ADA. Originally published elsewhere,[35,36,37] this model continues to expand toward a goal of providing a complete and defensive methodology for determining fitness for duty.

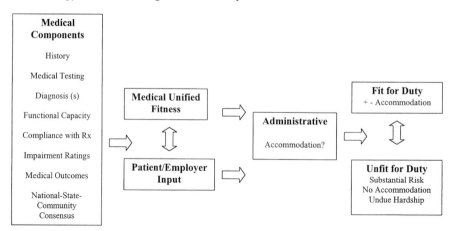

FIGURE 2.   Fitness for duty components.

TABLE 1. Twenty-one Different Categories of Health Concerns

Musculoskeletal—Upper Ext	Cardiovascular	Diabetes
Musculoskeletal—Hand	Hematology/Immunology/	Dermatology
Musculoskeletal—Leg	Oncology	Memory/Learning/Communication
Musculoskeletal—Spine	Ophthalmology	Psychiatric/Psychological/Emotional
Neurology—General	Otolaryngology	Substance Use Disorder
Epilepsy/Other Episodic	Gastroenterology	General Medical
Disorders	Genitourinary (M or F)	General Surgical
Pulmonary	Genitourinary	
	(Women's Pregnancy)	

The categories were selected to follow, in general, the sequence used in the 4th edition of the American Medical Association's *Guides to the Evaluation of Permanent Impairment.*[27]

The UFR has four purposes:

1. To assist workers who develop health problems to return to the appropriate work they can do.
2. To assist those who have health problems and who have not worked to gain employment at tasks they can accomplish effectively.
3. To help employers by providing guidelines for appropriate levels of work as determined by the employee's health condition.
4. To offer employers suggestions as to possible accommodations to consider in determining if an employee might accomplish the essential functions of a job.

The term "unified fitness" was used to focus on what an individual *can* do, rather than on what he or she cannot do. While many of the functional ability categories are concerned with specialized capabilities, such as vision, hearing, and learning, others are related primarily to physical demands for lifting or carrying. For many years, the U.S. Department of Labor (DOL) and the Social Security Administration have classified all jobs into five levels of exertion and skill (Table 2).[38] The DOL model is widely accepted and used in making legal determinations of disability and fitness for duty. The UMA's medical specialists have severity indexed, as outlined by the DOL work profiles, each of the 21 different categories of health concerns. This categorization scheme, established by consensus, provides a uniform standard necessary to meet the ADA's direct threat definition of "reasonable medical judgment that relies on the most current medical knowledge and/or the best available evidence." Currently, 5-year outcome data from the Utah Drivers License Division, which uses a similar rating scheme, shows positive predictive value for most of the profile categories.[39] A profile severity

TABLE 2. United States Department of Labor Physical Demands Characteristics of Work Chart

Physical Demand Level	Occasional (0–33% of Workday)	Frequent (34–66% of Workday)	Constant (67–100% of Workday)	Typical Energy Required
Very Heavy	Over 100 lbs.	Over 50 lbs.	Over 20 lbs.	Over 7.5 METS
Heavy	100 lbs.	50 lbs.	20 lbs.	6.4–7.5 METS
Medium	50 lbs.	20 lbs.	10 lbs.	3.6–6.3 METS
Light	20 lbs.	10 lbs. and/or Walk/Stand/Push/ of Arm/Leg controls	Negligible Pull/Push of Arm/Leg controls while seated	2.20–3.5 METS
Sedentary	10 lbs.	Negligible	Negligible	1.5–2.1 METS

METS = metabolic energy expenditure equivalents

level 1 indicates no present or past limitation for that category of health concern, while level 10 indicates a condition in which work of any sort does not appear to be indicated (Table 3).

The UFR's unique value lies in assessing an individual when more than one medical condition simultaneously exits. The severity profile of each medical category is recorded, with the most severe profile level indicating the patient's maximum safe work capability. Limitations of the musculoskeletal category profiles have been identified as not being specific enough, for which there continues to be ongoing updates and improvements. Since the 21 categories of health concerns involve comprehensive medical knowledge, the final fitness-for-duty statement should be made by a doctor of medicine or osteopathy, with input from the patient and other sources as indicated. The medical disposition should be limited to advising the employer about an individual's current functional abilities and limitations in relation to essential job functions and about whether the individual meets the employer's health and safety requirements.[40]

Final Fitness for Duty Statements: Interaction of Three Specific Functions

Unified fitness evaluation. In arriving at a final, defensible fitness statement, a number of contributing variables, including the history and physical examination, medical testing results, diagnosis, functional capacity evaluations, compliance with treatment guidelines, and medical outcome studies may need to be considered. After consideration of these components, a report is generated based on the intended use of the UFR (see end of chapter for information on obtaining form). Physicians have found the report form quick and easy to use. An "x" placed in the appropriate severity profile of each medical category and notations as to times and stability are sufficient. As recovery occurs, a simple change in the profile level allows additional work activity. There is room to add additional comments in unusual circumstances. In more complex cases or in special situations, a full profile of all categories may be needed.

Patient/employee function. After completion of the UFR by the physician, the patient takes (or sends) it to his or her employer and counsels with the company as to how the employer can best accommodate to the limitations recommended.

Employer functions. In response to the UFR suggesting appropriate capability because of an employee's health problem, the employer can use this information to make an appropriate work fitness-for-duty assessment. The employer also may use the suggested ideas for possible accommodations to help determine whether the essential functions of a job can be accomplished. This will help the employer materially in meeting their responsibilities under the ADA.

The UFR has no coercive or controlling effect, but is useful for employers to consider. A summary of the 21 health categories, along with the fitness profile levels,

TABLE 3.   Profile Severity Levels

1 = No problems
2 = Some problem, with complete recovery
3 = Mild
4 = Slight
5 = Moderate
6 = Severe
7 = Very severe
8 = Special considerations
9 = Under evaluation, temporary
10 = No work, permanent or during recovery

Profile Levels — notes for upper levels (columns 8–10):
- Level 8: According to special circumstances — depends upon nature of problem
- Level 9: Temporary adjustment — under evaluation — depends on situation
- Level 10: No work activity appropriate

Levels 1–2 (Neurology rows): All work activities

Code	Category	3	4	5	6	7
A-U	Musculoskeletal — Upper Extremity	Infrequent heavy lifting — affected extremity	Medium lifting — affected extremity	Light lifting — affected extremity	No lifting — affected extremity	No lifting — either extremity
A-H	Musculoskeletal — Hand	Minimal loss of skill/lifting — one hand	Slight loss of skill/lifting — one hand	Medium skill/lifting — one hand	Minimum skill/light tasks — bilateral	Substitute for all hand functions
A-L	Musculoskeletal — Lower Extremity	Heavy: May Lift — Occasional - 100 lbs. Frequent - 50 lbs. Constant - 20 lbs.	Medium: May Lift: Occasional - 50 lbs. Frequent - 20 lbs. Constant - 10 lbs.	Light: May Lift: Occasional - 20 lbs. Frequent - 10 lbs. Constant - Negligible	Sedentary: May Lift - Occasional - 10 lbs. Frequent - Negligible Constant - Negligible	Limited sedentary
A-S	Musculoskeletal — Spine					Limited sedentary
B-G	Neurology — General				Limited tasks or sedentary	Limited sedentary or substitute functions
B-E	Epilepsy/Other Episodic Disorders	Moderately high risk tasks	Moderate risk tasks	Slight risk tasks	Slight risk or special limits	Sedentary or ground-level tasks
C	Pulmonary (Lung)	Heavy, not sustained	Medium	Light or intermittent medium	Sedentary, without oxygen	Sedentary, with oxygen
D	Cardiovascular (Heart/Blood Vessels)	Heavy	Medium	Light	Sedentary	No risk to others
E	Hematology/Immunology/Oncology	Heavy	Medium	Light	Sedentary or decreased standing	Limited sedentary
F	Ophthalmology (Eye)	No commercial driving	No undue risk - moving equipment/power tools	Desk/bench work	Sound/light signals	No allergens/irritants
G	Otolaryngology (E.N.T.)	No special hearing skills	Limited hearing	No bearing required	Limit noise exposure	No allergens/irritants
H	Gastroenterology (Digestive)	Heavy, except at intervals	Medium	Medium — less work load	Sedentary	Selected facilities
I-G	Genitourinary - General (G.U.– Male or Female)	Heavy	Medium	Light	Sedentary	Selected facilities
I-W	Genitourinary — Women/Pregnancy	Heavy	Heavy, with adjustment	Medium	Light	Sedentary
J	Diabetes	Heavy	Heavy, with injections	Minimal risk tasks	Limited risk tasks	Sedentary/limit standing
K	Dermatology (Skin)	Limit exposure to allergens/irritants	Minimize irritants	Eliminate allergens	No exposure to irritants	No exposure to allergens
L-M	Memory/Learning/Communication	Learn new, complex tasks	Complex tasks; usual supervision	Previous complex tasks with assistance	New, simple tasks with supervision	Simple tasks with supervision
L-P	Psychiatric/Psychological/Emotional	All — with monitoring	Select tasks; monitoring	Medium tasks; close supervision	Limited tasks/risks; close supervision	Highly selected tasks/risks; close supervision
L-S	Substance Use Disorders	Moderately high risk tasks; normal supervision[a]	Moderate risk tasks; intermediate supervision[a]	Slight risk tasks; increased supervision[a]	Limited risk tasks; close supervision[a]	No risk to self; close supervision[a]
M-M	General Medical	Heavy; may reduce hours	Medium	Light	Sedentary	Limit exposure to others
M-S	General Surgery	Heavy; may reduce hours	Medium	Light	Sedentary	Depends on type of problem

Note (Diabetes): Allowance for access to snacks/meals and regular work schedules

FIGURE 3. Summary of profile levels and work activity

are found on the back of the report form (Fig. 3). Further detailed information on each of the 21 health categories is provided in the UFR booklet. A summary of the Musculoskeletal Spine section of the UFR booklet is presented below (Table 4).

CATEGORY: MUSCULOSKELETAL SPINE

Most people report low back problems at some time in their lives, and national statistics indicate a general yearly prevalence in the U.S. population of 15–20%.[41] Low back problems are the second most common symptomatic reason expressed by patients for office visits to primary care physicians.[42] Among working-age people surveyed, 50% admit to back symptoms each year,[43,44] and back symptoms are the most common cause of disability for persons under age 45.[45] Various estimates of the total annual societal cost of back pain in the United States range from $20 to $50 billion.[46] In most instances, individuals appear to accept or tolerate back pain as an expected part of life, especially as they become older. However, when the spine is injured, there may be clear indication for adjustments in work expectations.

The issue is of concern not only for the worker's comfort and efficiency, but for the possible effects of work activities in causing increased pathology. While the details of medical history, physical examination, and special tests are essential for a correct diagnosis, clinical experience and, possibly, a functional capacity assessment can be used to estimate a person's fitness in the workplace.

The spine is divided into three segments: cervical, thoracic, and lumbosacral. Each of the segments shares, in general, limits on weightbearing or posture, such as lifting, carrying, bending, reaching, and standing. Problems including the pelvis should be handled as related to the lumbosacral spine or as a special situation, depending on the circumstance. Hip problems are considered under Category A-L (musculoskeletal—lower extremity).

Fractures of any segment of the spine or spinal surgery usually requires a variable amount of time off work, followed by a return to work with limitations of lifting and car-

TABLE 4. Category: Musculoskeletal-Spine

Profile Level	Circumstances	Appropriate Work Activity*	Possible Accommodations
1	No past limitation	All	None
2	Past limitation fully recovered	All	None
3	Mild limitation of function, but with little likelihood of aggravation.	Heavy	None
4	Slight limitation of function and/or with slight risk of aggravation.	Medium	Use of assistive devices, minimize standing, limitation of lifting,
5	Moderate limitation of function and/or moderate risk of aggravation.	Light	bending, stooping, carrying, etc. Change in height of work surfaces.
6	Severe limitation of function and/or marked risk of aggravation.	Sedentary	Special equipment. Limit distance from vehicle to work site.
7	Very severe limitation of activities with pain and decreased stamina.	Sedentary, with limitations	Special equipment, limited hours, special schedules, rest periods, etc.
8	Special circumstances	Depending on specific problem	According to situation
9	Under evaluation	Depending on situation	Temporary adjustment
10	Health problem where work activity is inappropriate	None	Review if improved

*Profiles to be based on function with use of appropriate braces, etc.

rying even if protected by a brace or cast. Soft tissue lesions, on the other hand, usually become stabilized within a few weeks and generally permit a return to work with appropriate accommodations. As further healing takes place, the profile level and duration of exposure may be upgraded to permit more demanding work, bearing in mind the balance between the desire to return to a previous job versus the risk of aggravating the condition. Some degree of discomfort should be expected on return to work, even with appropriate accommodations. Chronic pain that extends beyond what might be expected from the defined pathology should be considered for its emotional overtones and also may be profiled under the psychiatric/psychological/emotional section, if appropriate.

If spinal injury results in significant damage to the spinal cord, causing partial or complete paraplegia, this condition also should be profiled under the general neurology section. If radiculopathy results, the effect on function of the limbs also may be profiled under the musculoskeletal—upper extremity section or the musculoskeletal—lower extremity section or both. If the cauda equina is damaged, bladder symptoms may be profiled under genitourinary and bowel symptoms under gastroenterology.

The following are some examples of suggested profile levels:
- A 22-year-old male with symptoms of neck and shoulder pain, normal clinical findings, with full range of motion; x-rays normal; Profile Level 3 with duration specified.
- A 30-year-old male with low back pain after a heavy load that he was helping to carry shifted; examination and x-rays negative; symptoms stabilized in 3 weeks; Profile Level 4, full-time.
- A 55-year-old female with a long history of low back pain treatments, with radiating leg pain (radiculopathy); decreased range of spinal motion; x-rays showed moderate spondylolysis and disc herniation at L5; Profile Level 5, duration specified.
- A 40-year-old obese male with gradual onset of mid-back pain after long hours of heavy lifting; extensive degenerative changes in the lumbar spine; Profile Level 4, duration specified.

These profiles are both dynamic and flexible. If a patient shows progressive recovery, worsening, or the development of another condition, the profile level, along with the exposure duration, can be modified as needed. For example, if the 55-year-old female patient above had a seizure 2 months ago, and was now on medication, she would currently have a profile level 7 under the epilepsy category and a level 5 under musculoskeletal-spine. These recommendations would suggest that her appropriate work activities would be "sedentary and ground level; using handheld tools with permitted exceptions."

History of Medical Condition

The medical history is one of the most important factors a physician or employer can rely on to identify worker's risk to themselves or others. The rationale for this recommendation is based on the medical literature.[47] For conditions such as low back pain (LBP), some believe that history is the most important component for the prediction of risk.[48,49] Recurrent episodes of LBP appear frequently to be a precursor of future LBP. Rowe[50] found that 83% of those with LBP had recurrent attacks. Patients with sciatica had a recurrence rate of 75%[51] Similar recurrence rates have been reported by other investigators.[52,53] In determining the significance of the history, a number of factors must be considered. These include; ongoing treatment, the number of visits received for an injury to the same region, prior objective testing to the same region, prior work restrictions because of problems in the same area, the duration since last episode, the number of prior episodes in the same region, and prior time lost from work because of symptoms in the same region.

These factors have been severity indexed (Fig. 4), which allows an evaluator a reasonable and logical approach to improve uniformity and reliability in determining risk from prior occurrences. Determining severity of prior occurrences, combined with other tests, may be a way of increasing the predictive value. Further outcome studies must be completed to refine and validate this process.

Functional Capacity Evaluations

The Functional Capacity Evaluation (FCE) is another component to assist in placing an individual in a UFR Profile. It is an extensive set of tests that purports to assess an individual's ability to perform work at the present and in the future.[54] A review of the medical literature on FCEs reveals that professionals who conduct, report, and interpret FCEs are concerned about the absence of formal standards, outcomes, and specific guidelines for these assessments. The ways in which the FCEs currently test for information vary in the number of measurements obtained, degree of standardization, clarity of the concepts and underlying theories, variety in choice of measuring instruments, adequacy of measurement for certain injury groups, use and availability of normative data, and ability to predict return to work or recurrence of injury.

Severity Indexing for Determining Future Risk			
Severity Index the History for Treatment/Testing to the Same Anatomical Region by the Following Schedule:			
Score	0	1pt.	2pts.
A Time Lost from Work in the Last 12 Months Because of Symptoms in the Same Region.	0	1-3 days	>3 days
B Number of Prior Episodes in the Same Region	0	1-3	>3
C Duration since Last Episode	0	1-3 Years	<1year
D Prior Work Restrictions Because of Problems in the Same Region	None	Temporary	Permanent
E Prior Objective Testing to the Same Region: (EMG-NCV, X-ray, MRI-CT, Bone Scan)	>3yrs	If taken prior to 2 years	If taken within the last 2 years
F Prior to latest claim, what ongoing Medical, Physical Therapy Chiropractor, etc, visits were received for an injury to the same region.	0 -2 times in last 3 yrs	3-6 times in last 3 yrs	>6 in last 3 yrs

Points	Risk	Recommendations
0 – 3 pts	Minimal Risk for Future Recurrence	
3 – 6 pts	Moderate Risk for Future Recurrence	Administrative or ergonomic/engineering considerations to reduce future risk of recurrence
>7 pts	High Risk for Future Reoccurrence	Individual being evaluated should not return to work at prior work level or forces
Total pts		

FIGURE 4. Prior history severity indexing and recommendations. A significant predictor of future problems in any given area is the patient's past medical history. This model provides a reasonable and logical approach for an evaluator to improve uniformity and reliability in determining risk from prior occurrences.

An extensive review of the 10 most used FCEs was published in the official journal of the American Physical Therapy Association.[55] Issues of interrater reliability, intrarater reliability, report writing, qualifications of examiners, examiner training, projection of findings to an 8-hour day, and safety demonstrate significant variations among systems manufacturers. Predictive validity is defined as the ability of any test to predict future performance. FCEs typically are ordered to assess current patient ability or future risk. Of the 10 most common commercially available systems, only one had any validation studies published in a peer-reviewed scientific journal. Regarding validity, the review article concludes, "Lack of peer-reviewed publications for the FCEs reporting the completion of validity studies leaves open the question of whether the FCEs are acceptable. With the exception of the PWPE (ErgoScience), the FCEs reviewed for this article do not provide the validly studies that are seen as the prerequisite for demonstrating that a measure is credible."[56] In summary, the FCE is not a stand-alone test, but currently a somewhat subjective test, that can be utilized with other findings, albeit with caution, in determining a fitness profile.

Worker Improvement Efforts

An essential component to be considered before placing an individual in a UFR profile is the effort the individual has expended to improve his or her health. Studies have demonstrated compensation for injuries can inherently affect effort and thereby prolong recovery,[57,58,59] increase disability,[60,61,62,63] and decrease the potential to return to work.[64,65,66] All individuals being considered for placement in a UFR profile, can be categorized into one of four effort quadrants (Fig. 5).

Considerable concern and resources are spent in determining the effort quadrant in which patients perform. Patients whose efforts are not sincere during rehabilitation or testing may overuse treatment, have a prolonged recovery, have increased cost of care, or receive unwarranted disability payments.[67,68,69] However, healthcare providers have been known to erroneously label patients as giving poor effort or as "symptom magnifiers." These unwarranted labels can be emotionally and financially devastating to the patient, particularly when an undiagnosed medical condition is discovered that was significantly limiting performance.

Currently, a number of procedures are promoted as ways a clinician can detect effort. An excellent and comprehensive review of the eight most widely used methods used to detect sincerity of effort is available (Table 5).[70] The article concludes: "The American Physical Therapy Association standards for measurements and practice require that clinical measurements used to detect sincerity of effort have established validity. Currently, clinicians do not have legitimate tools or methods with which to make these assessments. Any statements regarding sincerity of effort, therefore, are strictly clinical opinion. Therapists who draw unwarranted conclusions from test results are violating the rights of the person being tested." As with the conditioning of any athlete, effort assessments are best made by a clinician who has continuously worked with an

1. Can do Good Effort	3. Can't do Good Effort
2. Can Do Poor Effort	4. Can't Do Poor Effort

FIGURE 5. Effort quadrants.

TABLE 5.   Widely Used Methods for Determining Sincerity of Effort.

Waddell's nonorganic signs
Coefficient of variation
Bell-shaped curve
Rapid exchange grip
Correlation between musculosketal evaluation and functional capacity evaluation
Documentation of pain behaviors
Documentation of symptom magnification
Ratio of heart rate to pain intensity

individual over the course of rehabilitation. Even for a single visit, documentation of compliance, physiological observations, performance indicators, pain behaviors, and the therapist's intuition[71] are easy to record and provide the reader with an indication of the perceived effort individuals are expending to help themselves. A list of some of these indicators is given the acronym BICEPS (Fig. 6). Validation of these indicators will need to be prospectively studied.

Confidentiality of Information

Physicians and employers alike must remember that all medically related information must be kept confidential at the worksite and limited only to what is necessary for an appropriate job assignment or for making a reasonable job accommoda-

Individual Effort Indicators (BICEPS)		
Behavior	Compared with other patients having similar conditions, pain behaviors that appear amplified such as grimacing, verbal expression, over reaction, give away weakness, and non physiological pain and movement patterns should be noted during each visit.	
Intuition	Most clinicians have extensive experience as they have participated in the rehabilitation of hundreds of various individuals with different diagnosis. This valuable experience provides clinicians with an intuitive sense of an individuals desire to improve that is reportable.	
Compliance	Attendance	Number visits Scheduled/No. Attended.
	Punctuality	Time Scheduled /Time Began
	Completion of Program	Record % of Assigned Program to % Completed
Expectations:	Positive as well as negative comments reflecting personal expectation rehabilitation/Testing	"I have to get back to work", "When can I get back to work" etc. "I can't go back" or "I don't know why they are doing this to me, they know I will never be able to go back to work" etc.
Performance	Is the patient's observed performance consistent with what they indicate they can do?	Walking Tolerance
		Sitting Tolerance
		Standing Tolerance
Signs	Notes taken of the following physiological signs as to whether observations are consistent with experience with other patients with similar conditions.	Heart Rate:
		Respiration Rate
		Perspiration

FIGURE 6.

tion. In certain instances, an employer may have a "need to know" as described below. However, specific information about the nature of the medical condition must be kept confidential in the employee's personal medical record. Supervisors are only entitled to know the limitations of the profile level indicated. By using the UFR form and simply noting the nature of a worker's problem and checking the appropriate profile level, the ADA requirements for confidentiality are met and the employer is permitted to act in a prudent and reasonable fashion. Exceptions to this include the following: (1) supervisors and management must be informed about necessary work restrictions; (2) first aid and safety personnel should be informed if the disability may require emergency treatment or if any specific procedures are needed in the case of fire or other evacuations; (3) government officials can investigate compliance with ADA; (4) relevant information must be provided to state workers' compensation offices or second-injury funds; and (5) relevant information must be provided to insurance companies for cases in which the company requires a medical examination in order for health or life insurance to be provided.

Use of Skill and Judgment

The following quotation from the AMA Guides represents the philosophy by which use of the UFRs in the workplace should be governed:

The physician's judgment and his or her experience, training, skill, and thoroughness in examining the patient and applying the findings to the AMA Guides criteria will be factors in estimating the degree of the patient's impairment. These attributes comprise part of the art of medicine, which, together with a foundation in science, constitute the essence of medical practice. The evaluator should understand that other considerations will also apply, such as the sensitivity, specificity, accuracy, reproducibility, and interpretations of laboratory tests and clinical procedures, and variability among observers' interpretations of the test and procedures.[72]

SUMMARY

UFRs have been developed to enhance the objective flow of fitness-for-duty information between physicians and employers of any condition(s) physicians are presented with. These efforts are preliminary to what could become a more refined and objective method of describing individual fitness. UFRs also provide a service consistent with Principle VH of the American Medical Association's Principles of Medical Ethics, which states that, "a physician shall recognize a responsibility to participate in activities contributing to and improving the community."

Copies of the *Unified Fitness Report Booklet* and the Report Forms will be available at a reasonable cost from the Utah State Department of Health, 288 North 1460 West, P.O. Box 15680, Salt Lake City, Utah 84116-1580. All or part of the *United Fitness Report* Booklet may be duplicated freely by individuals or organizations for their use, but not for purposes of sale or profit.

Acknowledgment

Special acknowledgment is given to Dr. Madison Thomas, Task Force Chairman, and the 28 members of the Utah Medical Association who contributed to the UFR.

REFERENCES
1. Yelin E. Displaced concern: the social context of the work disability problem. Millbank Mem Fund Q. 1989;67(suppl 2, pt 1);114–166.
2. Leigh JP, Markowitz SB, Fahs M, Shin C, Landrigan PJ. Occupational injury and illness in the United States: estimates of costs, morbidity, and rnortality (see comments). Arch Intern Med. 1997;157:1557–1568.

3. State of Washington Department of Labor and Industries, Attending Doctor's Handbook, 1996, p4.

4. Harris L and Associates. Disabled Americans' Self Perceptions: Bringing Disabled Americans Into the Mainstream. New York:Harris&Associates; 1986

5. LaPlante MP. The demographics of disability: the Americans with disabilities act—from policy to practice. Milbank Mem Fund Q. 1991;69(suppl 1, pt 2):55–57.

6. Americans with Disabilities Act 42 USC, §12101 (1991).

7. Nagi S. An epidemiology of disability among adults in the United States. Milbank Mem Fund Q. 1976;54:439–468.

8. Yuker HE. The Disability Hierarchies: Comparative Reactions to Various Types of Physical and Mental Disabilities. Hempstead, NY: Hofstra University Press; 1987.

9. Berkowitz E. Disabled Policy: American's Programs for the Handicapped. New York:Cambridge University Press; 1987.

10. Stone D. The Disabled State. Philadelphia: Temple University Press; 1984.

11. Postal L. Medical-Legal Interference: Disability Evaluation. St. Louis, MO: American Medical Association; 1996:59.

12. Panzarella, JP, The nature of work, job loss, and the diagnostic complexities of the psychologically injured worker. Psych Ann 1991:21:10–15

13. Dent GL.Curing the disabling effects of employee injury. Risk Manage. 1985; January:30.

14 Derebery VJ, Tullis WH. Delayed recovery in the patient with a work compensable injury. J Occup Med 1983;25:829–835.

15. Nachemson AL. Work for all. Clin Orthop. 1983;179:77.

16. Mayer TG, Gatchel RJ, Kishono N. et al. Objective assessment of spine function following industrial injury: a prospective study with comparison group and one year follow up. Spine. 1985;10:483–493.

17. Dworkin RH, Handlin DS, Richlin DM, Brand L Vannucci C Unraveling the effects of compensation, litigation, and employment on treatment response in chronic pain. Pain. 1985;23:49–59.

18 Stung JP. The chronic disability syndrome. In: Aronoff GM, ed. Evaluation and Treatment of Chronic Pain. Baltimore, MD: Urban & Schwarzenberg; 1985.

19 Walton M. Thc Demming Management Method. New York: Putnam; 1986.

20. Gice J. Tomokins K. Cutting costs with return to work programs. Risk Manage. 1988;35:62–65.

21. Taylor T. Working around workers' injuries. Nation's Business. 1988;76:39–40.

22. Americans with Disabilities Act 42 USC § 12101 (1991).

23. Americans with Disabilities Act 42 USC § 12101 (1991).

24. Americans with Disabilities Act 42 USC § 12101 (1991).

25. Equal Opportunity Commission. Cumulative ADA Charge Data, March 31, 1996. Data compiled by the Office of Program Operations from the EEOC's Charge Data System's National Data Base.

26. Bell, C, Overview of the American with disability act and the family and medical leave act, Disability Evaluation, American Medical Association , Mosby St. Louis, Mo 1996 pp.582–591

27. Americans with Disabilities Act 26.42 U.S.C. § 12113(b); 29 C.F.R. § 1630.15(b)(2).

28. Thc Guides to the Evaluation of Permanent Impairment, 4th ed. Chicago, IL: American Medical Association; 1993.

29. A Technical Assistance Manual on the Employment Provision (Title I) of the Americans with Disabilities Act. Washington, DC: US Equal Employment Opportunity Commission; 1992:Section Vl-7.

30. Americans with Disabilities Act 42 USC § 12101 (1991).

31. Americans with Disabilities Act 42 USC § 12101 (1991).

32. A Technical Assistance Manual on the Employment Provision (Title I) of the Americans with Disabilities Act. Washington, DC: US Equal Employment Opportunity Commission; 1992:Section Vl-7.

33. A Technical Assistance Manual on the Employment Provision (Title I) of the Americans with Disabilities Act. Washington, DC: US Equal Employment Opportunity Commission; 1992:Section Vl-7.

34. Thomas MH. Work place Functional Ability Guidelines. Salt Lake City, UT: Utah Medical Association; 1994.

35. Johns RE Jr, Elegante JM, Teynor PD, et al: Fitness for duty. In Demeter S (ed): Disability Evaluation. American Medical Association, Mosby St. Louis, Mo 1996 pp 592–604

36. Johns RE Jr, Bloswick DS, Elegante JM, Chronic, recurrent low back pain, a methodology or analyzing fitness for duty and managing risk under the Americans with disability act. JOM Vol 36, no 5 may 1994.

37. Colledge AL, Johns RE Jr, Thomas MH. Functional abilities assessment: Guidelines for the workplace. JOEM. 1999;vol 41, no 3, Mar 1999;172–180.

38. United States Employment Service Dictionary of Occupational Titles, 4th ed. Washington, DC: US Government Printing Office; 1991:1013.

39. Diller E. Evaluating the existing system of drivers with medical conditions in Utah, Mountain injury control research center, University of Utah, 4–22-99.

40. Americans with Disabilities Act 42 USC § 12101 (1991).

41. Andersson GBJ. The epidemiology of spinal disorders. In: Frymoyer JW, editor. The adult spine: principles and practice.New York: Raven Press, Ltd.;1991. p.107–46.
42. Cypress BK. Characteristics of physician visits for back symptoms: A national perspective. Am J Public Health 1983 Apr;73(4):389–95.
43. Vällfors B. Acute, subacute and chronic low back pain: Clinical symptoms, absenteeism and working environment.Scand J Rehab Med Suppl 1985;11:1–98.
44. Sternbach RA. Survey of pain in the United States: The Nuprin pain report. Clin J Pain 1986; 2(1):49–53.
45. Cunningham LS, Kelsey JL. Epidemiology of musculoskeletal impairments and associated disability. Am J Public Health 1984;74:574–9.
46. Nachemson AL. Newest knowledge of low back pain. A critical look. Clin Orthop 1992;279:8–20.
47. RE Johns, Bloswick DS, Elegante JM, Chronic, recurrent low back pain, a methodology or analyzing fitness for duty and managing risk under the Americans with disability act. JOM Vol 36, no 5 may 1994.
48. Glover JR. Prevention of back pain. In: Jayson M, ed. The Lumbar Spine and Back Pain, 2nd ed. Tunbridge Wells, England: Pitman Medical; 1980.
49. Taylor PJ. Personal factors associated with sickness absence. A study of 194 men with contrasting sickness absence experience in a refinery population. Br J Ind Med. 1968;25:106–118.
50. Rowe ML. Preliminary statistical study of low baek pain. J Occup Med. 1963; 5:336–341.
51. Nachemson AL. Back problems in childhood and adolescence (in Swedish). Lakartidningen 1968;65:2831–2842.
52. Troup JDG, Martin JW, Lloyd DCEF. Back pain in industry. A prospective survey.Spine. 1981;6: 61–69.
53. Pedersen PA. Prognostic indicators in low back pain. J R Coll Gen Pracr 1981; 31:209–216.
54. Suesterhaus M.P Orthopedic Physical Therapy, Functional Capacity Evaluation Study Course, Orthopedic Section, Am Physical Therapy Association, May 1998, pp 1–14.
55. King PM, Tuckwell N. Barrett TE. A critical review of functional capacity evaluations. Phys Ther. 1998;78:852–866.
56. King PM, Tuckwell N. Barrett TE. A critical review of functional capacity evaluations. Phys Ther. 1998;78:852–866.
57. Greenough CG, Fraser RD. The effect of compensation on recovery from low back injury. Spine 1989;14-.947–55.
58. Hunter SJ, Shaha S, Flint DF, etal. Predicting Return to work, A long term follow-up study of railroad workers after low back injuries. Spine 1998, Vol 23 No 21, pp 2319–2328.
59. Sander RA, Meyers JE. The relationship of disability to compensation status in railroad workers, Spine 1986;11:141–3
60. Guest GH, Drummond PD. E!ffect of compensation on emotional state and disability in chronic back pain. Pain 1992; 48:125–30.
61. Jamison RN, Matt DA, ParrisWCV. Effects of time, limited vs. unlimited compensation on pain behavior and treatment outcome in low back pain patients. J Psychosom Res 1988;32:277–83.
62. Leavitt F. The physical exertion factor in compensable work injuries; A hidden flaw in previous research. Spine 1992;17:307–10.
63. Milhous RL, Haugh LD, Frymoyer J'W, et al. Determinants of vocational disability in patients with low back pain. Arch Phys Med Rehabil 1989;70:589–93.
64. Fredrickson BE, Trief PM, Van Beveren P, Yuan HA, Baum G. Rehabilitation of the patients with chronic back pain: a search for outcome predictors. Spine 1988;3:351–3
65. Guck TP, Meilman PW, Skultery FK Dowd ET. Prediction of long-term outcome of multidisciplinary pain treatment. Ach of Phy Med and Rehabil 1986, 67 233–6.
66. Milhous RL, Haugh LD, Frymoyer J'W, et al. Determinants of vocational disability in patients with low back pain. Arch Phys Med Rehabil 1989;70:589–93.
67. King PM. Analysis of approaches to detection of sincerity of effort through grip strength measurement. Work. 1998;10:9–13.
68. Robinson ME, Geisser ME, Hanson CS, O'Conner PD. Detecting submaximal efforts in grip strength testing with the coefficient of variation. Journal of Occupational Rehabilitation. 1993;3:45–50.
69. Baker JC. Burden of proof in detection of submaximal effort. WORK. 1998;10:63–70.
70. Lechner D,Bradbury SF, Bradley LA. Detecting sincerity of effort: a summary of methods and approaches. Phy Ther. 1998;78:867–888.
71. Hazard RG. Isokinetic trunk and lifting strength measurements: Variability as an indicator of effort. Spine. 1988;13:54–57.
72. The Guides to the Evaluation of Permanent Impairment, 4th ed. Chicago, IL: American Medical Association; 1993.

LEON H. ENSALADA, MD, MPH

THE IMPORTANCE OF ILLNESS BEHAVIOR IN DISABILITY MANAGEMENT

From Leon Ensalada & Associates
Hendersonville, Tennessee

Reprint request to:
Leon H. Ensalada, MD, MPH
235 East Main Street
Suite 101
Hendersonville, TN 37075

A small percentage of occupational injuries and illnesses account for a large proportion of the cost of disability. There is no evidence to suggest that this is due to the severity of injury or illness. Just the opposite appears to be true. For example, in the state of Washington, less than 5% of total claims cost $883 million in 1993; however, these were claims in which there were no objective medical findings.[69] What accounts for this seeming anomaly? Failure to recognize, and consequently consider, the relationship of illness behavior to injury, illness, impairment, and disability drives the cost of disability. Illness behavior is related to both injury or illness and to impairment or disability, and may partially or completely explain apparent association of these states[23] (Fig. 1).

Illness behavior encompasses a broad range of circumstances from unconscious symptom exaggeration to psychiatric disorders and malingering, characterized by mistaken beliefs, refusal to consider alternative explanations of symptoms, misattribution of symptoms, falsification of information, fabrication of complaints, manufactured disease, and exaggeration for profit or revenge. This review provides basic information necessary to understand these complex issues. The discussion is divided into three sections: basic terms and definitions, syndromes characterized by abnormal illness behavior, and methods for detecting deception.

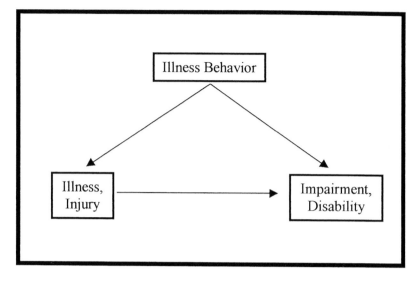

FIGURE 1.   The relationship of illness behavior to illness, injury, impairment, and disability. (From AMA: The Guides Newsletter. Washington DC, American Medical Association, May/June 1998; with permission.)

TERMS AND DEFINITIONS
Familiarity with the basic response styles provides a foundation for understanding the syndromes associated with deceptive behavior.

Basic Response Styles
1. **Honest responding** refers to a response style indicative of a patient's attempt to be accurate within his or her own frame of reference. Honest responding does not exclude nondeliberate distortion. Thus, factual inaccuracies must be evaluated in light of the patient's understanding and perceptions.
2. **Faking bad,** also known as *malingering, false imputation,* and *simulation,* refers to a response pattern in which there is an exaggeration or fabrication of symptoms and negative features, denial and/or minimization of positive traits, or misattribution of deficits to a false cause. Faking bad always involves looking more sick, dangerous, or negative than one is to accomplish some task or to obtain a desired outcome.
3. **Faking good,** also known as *defensiveness,* is the opposite of faking bad. It refers to a minimization and/or denial of symptoms and behaviors, an exaggeration or fabrication of positive points, or misattribution of blame to an outside source. Faking good always involves looking more attractive, healthier, or benign than one is to accomplish some task or to obtain a desired outcome.
4. **Invalidating** refers to a response style that attempts to render an evaluation meaningless.
5. **Hybrid responding** refers to any combination of the foregoing response styles. An example of hybrid responding drawn from occupational forensic evaluations is a report of outstanding capabilities (faking good) prior to an injury, followed by a report of substantial incapacity (faking bad) following an injury.

Dissimulation is a general term used to describe a person who is deliberately distorting and misrepresenting physical or psychological symptoms. Dissimulation may incorporate any response style with the exception of honest responding. **Distortion** refers to an intentional or unintentional misrepresentation of events. Unintentional distortion can be the consequence of various factors, including stress, recall problems, inattention, limited intelligence, physical disability, or mental illness.

Deception refers to inducing a false belief in another and is a conscious distortion of behaviors or self-report. It includes dissimulation and all other forms of dishonesty. **Misattribution** is the claim that a deficit is due to a false cause rather than the true cause; misattribution can be intentional or unintentional. **Unreliability** is a nonspecific term used to describe a response style that is not reliable, but in which no further clarification can be made with respect to intentionality.

Pure malingering, also known as *invention,* refers to the feigning of a disease when it does not exist at all in a particular patient. **Partial malingering** refers to the conscious *exaggeration* of existing symptoms or the fraudulent allegation that prior genuine symptoms are still present (also known as *perseveration*).

False imputation refers to the ascribing of actual symptoms to a cause consciously recognized to have no relationship to the symptoms. For example, authentic physical symptoms due to a clearly defined injury at home may be falsely attributed to a traumatic event at work.

Gradations of Response Styles

Gradations of distortion, which are important in addressing dispositional issues or making treatment recommendations, have been described.[54,55] In this scheme, the term malingering is reserved for cases where there is unequivocal evidence of deliberate dissimulation. In contradistinction, cases where intentionality is in doubt are characterized by two gradations of reliability.

1. **Self-report with limited reliability** occurs when the patient answers most of the questions with a fair degree of accuracy, but volunteers little and may distort or evade on circumscribed topics.
2. **Self-report without reliability** refers to a patient who, through exaggeration, convinces the clinician that his or her self-presentation is not accurate. Although malingering may be suspected, the patient's intent cannot be unequivocally established.
3. **Mild malingering** refers to unequivocal evidence that the patient is attempting to exaggerate, but the degree of distortion is minimal and plays only a minor role in the differential diagnosis.
4. **Moderate malingering** occurs when the patient, either through exaggeration or fabrication, attempts to present himself or herself as considerably more impaired than is the case. The distortions may be limited to either a few critical symptoms (for example, the fabrication of pain complaints) or may represent an array of lesser distortions.
5. **Severe malingering** occurs when the patient is extreme in his or her fabrication of symptoms to the point that the presentation is fantastic or preposterous.

SYNDROMES CHARACTERIZED BY ABNORMAL ILLNESS BEHAVIOR

Somatoform disorders, factitious disorders, malingering, and symptom magnification are clinical phenomena that lie along a continuum of abnormal illness behavior, from unconscious and unintentional processes to conscious and intentional ones.[53] These diagnostic categories represent various degrees of illness behavior characterized by the process of somatization. Somatization is a person's conscious or unconscious use of the body or bodily symptoms for psychological purposes or personal gain. Somatizing individuals are characterized by the propensity to experience and report somatic symptoms that have no pathophysiologic explanation, to misattribute them to disease, and to seek medical attention for them.[44] The prevalence of somatization varies according to the clinical setting and the medical specialty, but is reported to be 5–40% of patient visits.[28] Somatizing disorders result in an increased usage of medical services, significantly affecting the cost of medical care.[44] Conservative estimates indicate that at least 10% of all medical services are provided for patients who have no evidence of organic disease.[65]

Social and cultural forces can facilitate somatization. **Medicalization**—the invocation of a medical diagnosis to explain physical discomfort that is not caused by disease, and the application of a medical intervention to treat it—is one such influence in contemporary Western culture.[5] Furthermore, somatization is facilitated in cultures that accept physical disease for entry into the sick role, but reject psychological symptoms as an excuse for disability.[16]

Numerous **secondary gain** issues contribute to the development and process of somatization and abnormal illness behavior. Specific motivations for somatization include: manipulation of interpersonal relationships; privileges of the sick role, including sanctioned dependency; financial gain; communication of ideas or feelings that are somehow blocked from verbal expression; and the influence of interpsychic defense mechanisms.[27] The following reinforcers of inappropriate illness behavior are commonly encountered in the disability management setting: life structured around disability, treatment by multiple medical professionals, relief from occupational responsibilities, relief from household responsibilities, attention and support of spouse and family, relief from or assistance with parenting children, and the potential for financial compensation.[23]

A comparison of somatoform disorders, factitious disorders, malingering and symptom magnification syndrome is presented in Table 1. The features outlined in this table serve to facilitate the following discussion.

TABLE 1.   Somatoform Disorders, Factitious Disorders, Malingering, and Symptom Magnification Syndrome: Comparison of Features

	Symptoms for Gain	Deceptive State of Mind	Mental Disorder	DSM-IV Classification	ICD-9 Code	Rateable per *Guides*
Somatoform disorders	Yes	No	Yes	Yes	Yes	Yes
Factitious disorders	No	Yes	Yes	Yes	Yes	Yes
Malingering	Yes	Yes	No	Yes	Yes	No
Symptom magnification syndrome I. Refugee	Yes	No	No	No	No	No
Symptom magnification syndrome II. Game player	Yes	Yes	No	No	No	No
Symptom magnification syndrome III. Identified patient	No	Yes	No	No	No	No

From AMA: The Guides Newsletter. Washington DC, American Medical Association, May/June 1998; with permission.

Somatoform Disorders

Somatoform disorders are characterized by (1) physical complaints lacking a known organic basis or demonstrable physical findings, and (2) the presence of psychological factors judged to be etiologic or important in the initiation, exacerbation, or maintenance of the disturbance.[1] The common feature of somatoform disorders is the presence of physical symptoms that *suggest* a general medical condition (hence, the term somatoform), but which are *not fully explained* by a general medical condition, by the direct effects of a substance, or by another mental disorder. The symptoms must cause clinically significant distress or impairment in social, occupational, or other areas of functioning. In contrast to factitious disorders and malingering, the physical symptoms are **involuntary** and are not intentional. The DSM-IV describes seven somatoform disorders, two of which (conversion disorder and pain disorder) are particularly relevant to the arena of disability management.

The essential attribute of **somatoform conversion disorder** is the presence of symptoms or deficits affecting voluntary motor or sensory function that suggest a neurological or other general medical condition. Common examples of conversion symptoms include paralysis, abnormal movements, aphonia, blindness, deafness, or pseudoseizures. Conversion symptoms usually conform to a patient's concept of disease rather than to pathophysiologic mechanisms or anatomical patterns. Psychological factors are judged to be associated with the symptom or deficit based on the observation that the initiation of the symptom or deficit is preceded by conflicts or other stressors. The symptoms are not intentionally produced or feigned as in factitious disorder or malingering.

A diagnosis of conversion disorder relies on positive clinical findings clearly indicating that the symptom does not derive from organic disease, e.g., a demonstration of normal motor function in patients with "paralysis." A broad range of neurological conditions can be misdiagnosed as conversion disorder, including multiple sclerosis, myasthenia gravis, and idiopathic or substance-induced dystonias. The presence of a neurological condition, however, does not preclude a diagnosis of conversion disorder.

The essential feature of **somatoform pain disorder** is pain that is the predominate focus of the clinical presentation and is of sufficient severity to warrant clinical attention. The pain is associated with significant distress or impairment in social, occupational, or other important areas of functioning. Psychological factors are judged to play a significant role in the onset, severity, exacerbation, or maintenance of the pain. The prominent diagnostic attribute of the pain associated with psychological factors is preoccupation with pain and the absence of significant physical findings that might account for the pain or its intensity. Similar to conversion symptoms, the pain is manifested inconsistently with respect to known anatomic distribution; or, if it mimics a known disease entity, the pain cannot be adequately explained on the basis of any existing organic pathology. The pain symptoms are not intentionally produced or feigned as in factitious disorder or malingering.

Unlike the malingerer, the person with a somatoform disorder is ill. If the illness can be shown to be caused by a particular injury, it is compensable.

Factitious Disorders

Factitious disorders are somatizing states characterized by the **voluntary** production of signs, symptoms, or disease for no apparent goal other than to assume the patient role.[1,19,58] By contrast, the somatoform disorders are viewed collectively as having symptoms that are manifested unconsciously. A factitious illness is not real, genuine, or natural; the physical or psychological symptoms are controlled voluntarily, and clinical presentations are simulated to deceive the physician. The DSM-IV diagnostic criteria for factitious disorder include: "A. Intentional production or feigning of physical or psychological signs or symptoms. B. The motivation for the behavior is to assume the sick role. C. External incentives for the behavior (such as economic gain, avoiding legal responsibility, or improving physical well being as in malingering) are absent".[1] Factitious disorder subtypes are based upon the relative preponderance of psychological or physical symptoms. The DSM-IV requirement for evidence of internalized motivation is consistent with the notion that factitious disorders are *fundamentally a mental disorder.*[66]

Unfortunately, the DSM-IV provides no diagnostic standards for determining voluntariness (consciousness of actions) or intentionality (consciousness of motivation). The following criteria are recommended for determining the voluntary control of symptoms: (1) admission of deceit by the patient, (2) presence of physiologically impossible symptoms, (3) observable evidence, (4) symptoms contradicted by objective testing, (5) physical evidence, and (6) nonstereotypical response to treatment.[48] The determination of voluntariness does not establish intentionality; i.e., consciousness of actions and consciousness of motives are not necessarily related. For instance, a patient exhibiting a marked increase in pain behavior in the presence of an attentive and supportive spouse can be unaware of the association between his or her behavior (which is voluntary) and the behavior of the spouse (which is the motivation for the patient's behavior). The difficulties of diagnosing factitious disorders by DSM-IV criteria are clear: the physician must determine conscious production of symptoms, based upon unconscious motives, in a noncooperative patient.

Malingering

Malingering phenomena traditionally have been viewed as representative of conscious desires to obtain money or drugs, avoid work or prosecution, or evade undesirable duties.[6,8,11,43,54,56,57] The DSM-IV defines malingering as "the intentional production of false or grossly exaggerated physical or psychological symptoms motivated by external incentives such as avoiding military duty, avoiding work, obtaining financial compensation, evading criminal prosecution, or obtaining drugs," and allows that malingering may be socially adaptive in isolated circumstances, for example, "feigning illness while a captive of the enemy during war time."[1] The DSM-IV does not confer disease status to malingering; it is *not a mental disorder*. Rather, it is a condition "that may be a focus of clinical attention." Unfortunately, and similar to the problem encountered with the DSM-IV definition of factitious disorder, no guidance is provided for determining consciousness of actions (voluntariness) or consciousness of motivation (intentionality).

The DSM-IV model presupposes that malingering is likely to occur with (1) evaluations conducted for forensic purposes, (2) persons whose claims are discrepant with objective findings, (3) persons uncooperative with evaluation and treatment, and (4) persons diagnosed with antisocial personality disorder. These criteria are clinically inadequate for diagnosing malingering. First, they fail to distinguish distorting influences such as evaluation anxiety and fatigue from deliberate deception. Second, they emphasize exaggeration and fabrication of symptoms to the neglect of denial and defensiveness. Third, they associate deliberate deception with a personality type despite no proven association between antisocial personality disorder and malingering.[59] Fourth, malingerers are often highly cooperative, seek out treatment, and are willing to discuss or volunteer symptoms.[21]

Rogers assessed the efficacy of DSM-IV indicators of malingering on a forensic sample, and found that the use of two or more indicators as specified by DSM-IV proved ineffective at identifying malingerers.[56] Two-thirds of the malingerers were correctly identified by this criterion; however, for every malingerer correctly identified, nearly four times as many bona fide patients were mischaracterized as malingerers. These findings suggest that persons exceeding the DSM-IV criterion of two or more indicators have approximately a one in five chance of truly being a malingerer. Consequently, the clinical application of the DSM-IV indicators of malingering is not recommended.

Unintentional Distortion

Nondeliberate distortion of words or behavior is common and must be excluded prior to concluding that malingering has occurred. Unintentional distortion can be associated with evaluation anxiety, fatigue, limited intelligence, physical incapacity, inattention, memory problems, and mental disorders.[7] Failure to account for nondeliberate distortion renders conclusions regarding malingering invalid.

Symptom Magnification Syndrome

Symptom magnification syndrome (SMS), a concept introduced by Matheson to provide rehabilitation and vocational specialists with insight into patients' behavior, is defined as a "self-destructive, socially reinforced behavioral response pattern consisting of reports or displays of symptoms which function to control the life circumstances of the sufferer . . . it is a self-destructive pattern of behavior which is learned and maintained through social reinforcement. This pattern of behavior is composed of reports and/or displays of symptoms, the effect of which is to control the life circumstances of the sufferer."[46] Matheson acknowledges that SMS is not a psychiatric diagnosis, "although each of the SMS types has an analog in the psychiatric literature."[46]

Matheson identified three types of SMS. The **type I** symptom magnifier (the "refugee") is a person whose illness behavior provides an escape from an apparently unresolvable conflict or life situation. The analog to type I SMS in the DSM-IV is somatoform disorder. The **type II** symptom magnifier (the "game player") is a person who has discovered that his or her symptoms provide an opportunity for positive gain. The analog to type II SMS in the DSM-IV scheme is malingering. The **type III** symptom magnifier (the "identified patient") is a person whose symptoms ensure survival and maintenance of the patient role. The analog to type III SMS in the DSM-IV is factitious disorder.

SMS is a label for a type of illness behavior characterized by symptom exaggeration.[26,47] As a learned pattern of behavior, it can be unlearned; thus, it is not permanent, and it is not rateable per The American Medical Association's *Guides to the Evaluation of Permanent Impairment*, 4th edition.

DETECTING DECEPTION

Some frequently cited studies call into question clinicians' capacity to detect deception. In Rosenhahn's classic study, eight pseudopatients were admitted to psychiatric hospitals, all alleging that they heard atypical voices.[63] Although they stopped reporting symptoms once they were admitted, all were diagnosed as schizophrenic and remained hospitalized from 9 to 52 days, illustrating the inability of clinicians to identify feigned psychosis. More recent studies assessed the capacity of neuropsychologists to identify malingering when presented with only the raw data from neuropsychological tests and batteries. Heaton and colleagues found that neuropsychologists performed at best 20% above chance levels when attempting to distinguish persons faking dysfunction from genuine, nonlitigating patients with relatively severe brain injuries.[40] Worse yet, Faust and colleagues found that none of 42 neuropsychologists identified malingering after examining test profiles of children who were instructed to fake brain injury.[24,25]

Although the findings of Heaton and Faust are often interpreted to reveal clinicians' incapacity to detect malingering, the studies support a more limited conclusion; namely, clinicians perform poorly when attempting to detect deception using only information available from pencil-and-paper measures. In a more recent study, Trueblood and Binder found neuropsychologists to be highly accurate in distinguishing malingering from traumatic brain injury when informed that the study involved feigned cognitive deficits, consistent with the notion that poor performance in earlier studies was due in part to a failure to consider malingering in the differential diagnosis.[68] Furthermore, many persons faking or feigning a physical or mental disorder are expressing genuine distress regarding their current life circumstances. Clinicians arrive at an erroneous conclusion by equating the genuineness of this distress with the genuineness of the symptom presentation.

Any physical or psychiatric disorder can be exaggerated, faked or feigned.[15, 19,33,50,51,52,58] Although the methods for detecting deception vary depending on the claimed deficit, a **general approach** to identifying deception is based on: **(1)** evidence of consistency in the history or examination, **(2)** the likelihood that the set of symptoms the patient reports makes medical sense, i.e., fits a reasonable disease pattern, **(3)** an understanding of the patient's current situation, personal and social history, and emotional predispositions, **(4)** the emotional reactions to the symptoms, such as patients who appear comfortable while reporting significant distress, **(5)** standardized assessment instruments, and **(6)** tests of dissimulation, which can be employed with patients whose motivations or complaints are suspect.

The following sections describe some methods for detecting deception. The discussion is not comprehensive. For instance, a review of the detection of malingered neuropsychological deficits is beyond the scope of this article. Several reviews of assessing feigned neuropsychological impairment are available to the interested reader.[29,60]

History

The first major component of the history is what is learned absent the patient's self-report.[42] This information is obtained from medical records, employment records, school records, driving records, service records, and criminal records, and from interviews with family members, friends, teachers, or employers. The importance of obtaining information from corroborative sources cannot be overstated. The detection of false imputation and assessing issues of exacerbation or aggravation depend upon having access to this information.

The other major component of the history is the patient's self-report obtained during the patient's interview. Potential interview strategies for the assessment of deception have been described:[54]

- **Symptom subtlety:** Patients attempting to exaggerate exhibit a tendency to endorse more blatant than subtle symptoms.
- **Severity of symptoms:** Patients attempting to exaggerate endorse an unlikely number of symptoms with extreme or unbearable severity.
- **Rare symptoms:** Potential exaggerators often have difficulty distinguishing symptoms that are infrequent in patient populations from those that are more common. Consequently, such persons often endorse many rare symptoms.
- **Symptom onset and resolution:** Potential exaggerators may not be aware of the course of physical or mental disorders, and report either an unusually sudden onset or a resolution that is implausible given the nature of the purported disorder.

- **Improbable failure rate:** Even severely disturbed patients typically can complete simple cognitive tasks. Some patients feign substantial impairment on tasks that all but the most impaired individuals would accomplish.
- **Reported versus observed symptoms:** Persons attempting to exaggerate are often unaware of the incongruities between their actual presentation and reported impairment. This consists of easily observable behavior which may be documented by the physician. For example, following an injury, a truck driver reports an inability to sit for more than 5 minutes without excruciating pain, but he is observed to sit (apparently comfortably) for 60 minutes during the interview.
- **Clinical observations:** Patients attempting to exaggerate may exhibit important attitudinal variables; for example, an eagerness to discuss their symptoms, an elaboration of symptoms, or a theatrical quality to their presentation.
- **Consistency of symptoms:** Exaggerators often have difficulty remembering which symptoms they reported and their severity.
- **Selectivity of symptoms:** Some individuals attempting to exaggerate are not selective or are indiscriminate in their endorsement of physical problems.
- **Improbable or absurd symptoms:** This is an extension of the rare symptom category described previously. Improbable or absurd symptoms have a preposterous or fantastic quality, which makes them unlikely by definition to be true symptoms. For example, a self-report of "numbness" of the front half of the body is very unlikely to be an accurate reflection of a physical disorder. Waddell described "inappropriate" symptoms referable to nonspecific or mechanical low back pain, including tailbone pain, whole-leg pain, whole-leg numbness, whole-leg giving way, and no pain-free spells.[70,71]
- **Overly specified symptoms:** Persons attempting to exaggerate often endorse symptoms with a nonrealistic degree of precision.
- **Symptom combinations:** Patients attempting to exaggerate a physical or mental disorder are often unaware of which symptoms are likely or unlikely to coexist. With symptom combinations, the patient is asked whether he or she is experiencing several symptoms. Although commonly experienced individually, these symptoms rarely are present simultaneously.

Examination

Discerning discrepancies between the signs associated with a condition and the findings observed during the examination provides a basis for detecting deception, because feigned disorders appear to be modeled on a lay conceptualization of impairment that is often at variance with the features of actual disorders. For example, a pseudo-organic presentation of loss of sensation and weakness in an entire leg is common in exaggerators, although such symptoms in association with nonspecific low back pain are not ordinarily found in genuine patients. It follows that detecting deception during the examination requires a thorough knowledge of what is expected for the condition in question, and the capacity to observe or elicit what is expected and what is not.

In their classic studies of chronic low back pain, psychologic stress, and illness behavior, Waddell and colleagues were able to separate the standard signs of physical pathology and the inappropriate signs of illness behavior.[70,71] A group of eight inappropriate responses to physical examination in low back pain, divided into five categories, were found to form a homogeneous group of signs clearly separable from the standard signs of physical pathology. The common feature of all of the inappropriate signs was magnification, which was termed "magnified illness behavior." The authors pointed out, however, that the inappropriate signs did not exclude the presence of physical pathology and emphasized that isolated inappropriate signs were not clinically significant, suggesting a cutoff score of three or more signs.

Recently, Main and Waddell revisited the so-called Waddell's signs, emphasizing the following: (1) the inappropriate responses to physical examination in low back pain are not a substitute for a comprehensive psychological assessment but rather should be "understood as part of a wider set of pain behavior assessment tools such as pain drawings, reporting of behavioral symptoms, need for walking aids, and need for extended downtime," (2) differences among examiners "and the number of behavioral signs found may illustrate inconsistencies in the manner in which the signs are elicited, unwitting bias or even prejudice," and (3) the signs should not be misinterpreted as proof of malingering, explaining "in the absence of distress, fear, mistaken beliefs, maladaptive coping strategies, and active attempts to seek treatment, it is perhaps more likely that the signs are evidence of simulation, but the behavioral signs cannot be interpreted in isolation."[45]

Maximum Voluntary Effort Assessment

One of the most straightforward methods to measure maximum voluntary effort is based on the assumption that repetitive trials within a brief span of time are stable; that is, less than full effort over multiple trials yields increased **variability in performance.** Variability of performance can be assessed using the coefficient of variation, which is the standard deviation of a set of measurements divided by the mean of the set of measurements. The coefficient of variation is particularly useful in assessing the consistency of a person's performance during strength testing. Assuming that the equipment is properly calibrated and the test is performed correctly, a high coefficient of variation ($> 15–20\%$) is consistent with the patient's not having exerted a full effort. However, an increased coefficient of variation only reveals that the task was performed with less than maximum effort; clinicians must determine the person's motivation for the inconsistent performance from the total clinical context.

Additional techniques have been reported to help detect persons who exert less than maximal effort on grip-strength testing. Stokes reported that the plotting of **grip-strength measurements** from each of the five handle settings of a sealed hydraulic dynamometer would produce a bell-shaped curve, but persons not exerting maximum effort produce results yielding a straight line or flat curve.[67] Hildreth described an additional technique known as the rapid- exchange grip method for assessing submaximum effort on grip-strength testing.[41] In this protocol, after the dynamometer has been set to the position at which the patient had previously achieved maximal grip strength, the patient is instructed to rapidly alternate hands while gripping the dynamometer. If maximal performance has not been achieved on the static test, the rapid-exchange grip shows a significant increase in grip strength on the affected side. This technique is useful in differentiating the patient whose decreased performance is secondary to pain from those who voluntarily perform submaximally.

Minnesota Multiphasic Personality Inventory

The Minnesota Multiphasic Personality Inventory (MMPI) is the most widely used and researched objective personality inventory. The MMPI was published in 1943; a re-standardized version, the MMPI-2, was published in 1989. The MMPI-2 is an objective, actuarial-based instrument composed of 567 affirmative statements to which the individual provides a true or false response. Four previous validity scales (L, F, K, "cannot say"), along with three new validity scales (FB, TRIN, VRIN) provide an assessment of test validity and an assessment of two dichotomous test-taking attitudes; namely, malingering ("faking bad") and defensiveness ("faking good"). Raw scores are converted to uniform T-scores to allow easy comparison. Normal T-scores generally range from 50 to 65.

The MMPI validity scales assess the accuracy of item endorsement; that is, the validity scales verify whether a person has adopted a response set either to malinger or to be defensive.[2,3,4,36,61] The F-scale is one of the validity scales used to assess malingering, since its items were selected to detect unusual or atypical ways of endorsing. Elevations on the F-scale can occur due to inconsistent patterns of item endorsement, presence of actual psychopathology, and malingering. Thus, it is difficult to ascertain the reason for an elevation on the F-scale without considering other indicators of the consistency and accuracy of item endorsement. To illustrate, although a T-score greater than 100 on the F-scale does not reflect actual psychopathology, it could be consistent with either an inconsistent pattern of item endorsement or malingering. Hence, the F-scale is best used in conjunction with other validity indicators which distinguish between exaggerated MMPI profiles versus those selecting random responding.

Although MMPI measures of malingering are positively related to measures of psychopathology, elevations in the MMPI validity indices due to genuine disorders are modest, particularly with less severe conditions.[20] In addition, there are particular differences in clinical scale patterns between malingerers and those with genuine disorders. Empirical tables are available for comparing an examinee's MMPI results with those obtained by normal individuals, individuals with a disorder, and individuals instructed to simulate a disorder.[37,64] MMPI results can provide strong evidence of malingering when the items are endorsed consistently but inaccurately.

For the interested reader, a number of MMPI resources are available, including texts and interpretive manuals,[9,17,18,22,34,35,38] reviews of MMPI assessment of malingering,[29,37] and meta-analyses of malingering on the MMPI[10] and MMPI-2.[62]

Symptom Validity Testing

Symptom validity testing (SVT), also known as forced-choice testing, is an effective means of assessing the validity of sensory and memory deficits, including tactile anesthesias, paresthesias, blindness, color blindness, tunnel vision, blurry vision, and deafness.[12,13,14,30,31,39,49,50,51,52] The common feature among these symptoms is a claimed inability to perceive or remember a sensory signal. The adaptability of this technique to perceptual or memory complaints is likely limited only by the examiner's imagination. Unfortunately, symptom validity testing is not adaptable to evaluating claims of internal sensory signals, for example, pain.

Symptom validity testing is comprised of two elements: (1) a specific ability is assessed by a large number of items presented in a multiple-choice format, and (2) an examinee's performance is compared to the likelihood of success based on chance alone (i.e., no ability). Symptom validity tests usually have two multiple-choice alternatives; thus, the probability of purely guessing the correct response (i.e., analogous to no ability at all) is 50%. Scores significantly below chance performance indicate that the sensory cues must have been perceived, but the examinee chose not to report the correct answer; alternative explanations are not apparent.

A coin toss provides a familiar model to understand this technique. For example, a blind person does not have the capacity necessary to perceive the sensory cues required to call heads or tails correctly except at a chance rate. No scoring advantage is achieved by calling heads or tails in any pattern or order. Heads and tails are the only possible responses (two alternatives), and the task requires the examinee to make only one response (forced choice). In the case of total impairment, (i.e., total blindness),

TABLE 2.   Probabilities Associated with Number of Correct Responses in 100 Trials

Correct Responses	Z	p (one-tailed)
50	0.0	.5000
49	0.10	.4602
48	0.30	.3821
47	0.50	.3085
46	0.70	.2420
45	0.90	.1841
44	1.10	.1357
43	1.30	.1151
42	1.50	.0668
41	1.70	.0446
40	1.90	.0287
39	2.10	.0179
38	2.30	.0107
37	2.50	.0062
36	2.70	.0035
35	2.90	.0019

performance should approximate chance responding (50% accuracy with a two-choice task). A significant deviation from chance responding is defined as an accuracy score with a probability less than some specified level (for example, $p < 0.05$ or $p < 0.01$) as determined by the binomial probability distribution (Table 2). Specifically, the one-tailed probability of obtaining less than 40 correct responses in 100 trials with a two-choice task is less than 2% ($p < 0.0179$). Achieving less than 36 correct answers would occur by chance less than twice in a thousand tests ($p < 0.0019$).

The positive predictive value of the symptom validity technique is likely to be quite high, because there is no alternative explanation to deliberate distortion when performance is below the probability of chance. However, the sensitivity of this technique is not likely to be as good because many deceptive examinees do not claim a total deficit and, therefore, are not expected to perform significantly below chance levels. Moreover, some deceptive examinees violate the rules of the technique; for example, they avoid the signal cue, respond with a pattern, or repeat the same answer, which will ensure a 50% response rate. Consequently this technique is analogous to a thermometer: positive findings indicate that a problem is present, but negative findings do not rule out the problem.

Symptom validity testing provides an opportunity to show more than a low score. It demonstrates that the examinee performed below the probabilities of chance. Scoring below a norm can be explained in many different ways (e.g., fatigue, evaluation anxiety, inattention, intoxication, limited intelligence,), but scoring below the probabilities of chance alone has no alternative explanation. Scoring below the probabilities of chance is strong evidence of malingering; it provides strong evidence that the examinee received the sensory cues and denied the perception. Deceptive examinees miss the expected 50% accuracy for several reasons. First, the symptom validity technique confronts deceptive examinees quite directly, for it is difficult to maintain a properly randomized response pattern that will result in a score within the range of chance in 100 trials. Second, deceptive examinees assume that the impaired performance requires less than 50% accuracy. Deceptive examinees do worse than chance, because they intentionally suppress the correct answers on items to which they know the answers. However compelling the inference is that the examinee who scores below probabilities is deliberately motivated to perform poorly, the conclusion of malingering must be derived from the total clinical context.[32]

Alternative Explanations

Alternative explanations for the indicators of dissimulation must be considered because the greater the likelihood of an alternative explanation, the lower the positive predictive value. For example, rare symptoms are infrequently found in the patient population; the presence of several rare symptoms, although consistent with deliberate distortion, does not preclude other explanations. In contradistinction, a large number of rare symptoms or symptom combinations are extremely unlikely in bona fide patients. For example, regional weakness or sensory loss has been described to signify feigning. Alternative explanations include Axis I symptoms (e.g., somatoform conversion disorder) or Axis III symptomatology (e.g., a neurologic condition). Inclusion of these alternatives and the reasons why they are not compelling strengthen conclusions about dissimulation.

The indicators denoted in Table 3 are categorized into moderate, low, and no probability that such findings occur without dissimulation. The indicators in the moderate category may also be seen occasionally in honest, nondissimulating patients. Indicators in the low category have a very small probability of being observed. The indicators in the none category are not open to alternative explanations. Symptom validity testing scores significantly lower than chance performance indicate that the sensory cues must have been perceived, but the patient chose not to report the correct answer. Other viable explanations are not apparent. Similarly, quality surveillance information depicting a marked difference in a person's capacity in the community as compared to the person's capacity during a medical evaluation is not open to an alternative explanation.

When **assessing deception,** the recommendations of Wasyliw and Cavanaugh are pertinent. Evaluators should avoid: **(1)** blind testing and interpretation, (e.g., using a stock procedure regardless of the specifics or without review of prior history and evaluation), **(2)** lack of personality and psychopathology evaluation, **(3)** "gut" impressions of diagnosis or issues of malingering without clear objective or observational data, **(4)** conclusions as to organicity or malingering based on single tests, intelligence testing alone or performance on personality tests, **(5)** conclusions that loss or reduction in functioning has occurred without historical assessment of prior

TABLE 3.   Probability of Alternative Explanations

Moderate
Isolated, nonorganic sensory or motor signs
Mild to moderate elevations on MMPI validity scales
Rare symptoms
Sudden onset or resolution
Severity of symptoms
Nonselective reporting of symptoms
Dramatic presentation
Low
Multiple nonorganic sensory or motor signs
Marked elevations on MMPI validity scales
Inconsistent clinical presentation
Improbable or absurd symptoms
Contradictory symptoms
Unlikely symptom combinations
None
Symptom validity testing
Surveillance

functioning, **(6)** prognostic conclusions based on testing performed prior to maximum recovery, **(7)** conclusions as to degree of recovery based on the client's self-description alone, and **(8)** conclusions that deficits were due to a specific historical incident based on test data alone.[72]

SUMMARY

Recognizing the confounding effect of illness behavior on the relationship between injury or illness and impairment or disability is an essential component of disability management. The possibility of malingering must be addressed when financial issues or other external incentives are present. Although knowledge of conditions enables the clinician to make predictions about deficits from information about an injury or illness, the presence of an organic disorder does not exclude malingering. Likewise, the presence of malingering does not exclude an organic disorder.

The clinician must be able to distinguish unintentional distortion from deliberate deception and be able to recognize the wide range of circumstances in which distortion and deception play a role. Since distortion is not likely to be identified, no less characterized, during a diagnostic interview, the clinician must rely on information obtained from the diagnostic examination, medical and other relevant records, standardized assessment instruments, and on tests of dissimulation.

REFERENCES

1. American Psychiatric Association: Diagnostic and statistical manual of mental disorders, 4th ed. Washington, DC, APA, 1994.
2. Austin JS: The detection of fake good and fake bad on the MMPI-2. Ed Psychol Measure 52:669–674, 1992.
3. Bagby RM, Rogers R, Buis T: Detecting malingered and defensive responding on the MMPI-2 in a forensic inpatient sample. J Pers Assess 62:191–203, 1994.
4. Bagby RM, Rogers R, Buis T, Kalemba V: Malingered and defensive response styles on the MMPI-2: An examination of validity scales. Assessment 1:31–38, 1994.
5. Barsky AJ, Borus JF: Somatization and medicalization in the era of managed care. JAMA 274(24): 1931–1934, 1995.
6. Bash IY, Alpert M: The determination of malingering Ann NY Acad Sci 347:86–99, 1980.
7. Belli RF: Influences of misleading postevent information: Misinformation interference and acceptance. J Psychol 121:326–351, 1989.
8. Ben-Shakar G, Furedy JJ: Theories and applications in the detection of deception. New York, Springer-Verlang, 1990.
9. Berry DTR: Detecting distortion in forensic evaluations with the MMPI-2. In Ben-Porath YS, Graham JR, Hall GCN, Hirschman RD, Zaragoza M (eds): Forensic Application of the MMPI-2. Thousand Oaks, CA, Sage, 1995, pp 82–102.
10. Berry DTR, Baer RA, Harris MJ: Detection of malingering on the MMPI: A meta-analytic review. Clin Psychol Rev 11:585–598, 1991.
11. Berry DTR, Wetter MW, Baer RA: Assessment of malingering. In Butcher JN (ed): Clinical Personality Assessment: Practical Approaches. New York, Oxford University Press, 1995, pp 236–248.
12. Bickart WT, Meyer RG, Connell DK: The symptom validity technique as a measure of feigned short-term memory deficit. American J Forens Psychol 9:3–11, 1991.
13. Binder LM: Forced-choice testing provides evidence of malingering. Arch Phys Med Rehabil 72:377–380, 1992.
14. Binder LM, Pankratz L: Neuropsychological evidence of a factitious memory complaint. J Clin Exp Neuropsychol 9:167–171, 1987.
15. Boffeli TJ, Guze SB: The simulation of neurologic disease. Psychiatr Clin North Am 15:301–310, 1992.
16. Brodsky CM: Sociocultural and interactional influences on somatization. Psychosomatics 24:673–680, 1984.
17. Butcher JN, Dahlstrom WG, Graham JR, Tellegen A, Kaemmer B: MMPI-2: Manual for administration and scoring. Minneapolis, University of Minnesota Press, 1989.
18. Butcher JN, Williams CL: Essentials of MMPI-2 and MMPI-A interpretation. Minneapolis, University of Minnestoa Press, 1992.
19. Carlson RJ: Factitious psychiatric disorders: Diagnostic and etiologic consideration. Psychiatr Med 2:383–388, 1985.

20. Chaney HS, Cohn CK, Williams SG, Vincent KR: MMPI results: A comparison of trauma victims, psychogenic pain, and patients with organic disease. J Clin Psychol 40:1450–1454, 1984.
21. Cornell DG, Hawk GL: Clinical presentation of malingerers diagnosed by experience forensic psychologists. Law Human Behav 13:374–383, 1989.
22. Dahlstrom WG, Welsh GS, Dahlstrom LE: An MMPI handbook: Vol I: Clinical Interpretation. Rev ed. Minneapolis, University of Minnesota Press, 1972.
23. Ensalada LH: Illness behavior. In The Guides Newsletter. Washington DC, AMA, May/June 1998.
24. Faust D, Hart K, & Guilmette TJ: Pediatric malingering: The capacity of children to fake believable deficits of neuropsychological testing. J Consult Clin Psychol 56:578–582, 1988.
25. Faust D, Hart K, Guilmette TJ, Arkes HR: Neuropsychologists' capacity to detect adolescent malingerers. Prof Psychol: Research Pract 19:508–515, 1988.
26. Febrega H, Van Egeren L: The behavioral framework for the study of human disease. Ann Intern Med 84:200–208, 1976.
27. Ford CV: The somatizing disorders. Psychosomatics 27:327–337, 1986.
28. Ford CV: The Somatizing Disorders: Illness As a Way of Life. New York, Elsevier, 1983.
29. Franzen MD, Iverson GL, McCracken LM: The detection of malingering in neuropsychological assessment. Neurophysiol Review 1:247–279, 1990.
30. Frederick RI, Carter M, Powel J: Adapting symptom validity testing to evaluate suspicious complaints of amnesia in medicolegal evaluations. Bull Acad Psychiatr Law 23:231–237, 1995.
31. Frederick RI, Foster HG: Multiple measures of malingering on a force-choice test of cognitive ability. Psychol Assess: J Clin Consult Psychol 3:596–602, 1991.
32. Frederick RI, Sarfaty SD, Johnston JD, Powel J: Validation of a detector of response bias on a force-choice test of nonverbal ability. Neuropsychology 8:118–125, 1994.
33. Gorman WF: Neurological malingering. Behav Sci Law 2:67–73, 1984.
34. Graham JR: The MMPI: A practical guide, 2nd ed. New York, Oxford University Press, 1987.
35. Graham JR: MMPI-2: Assessing Personality and Psychopathology, 2nd ed. New York, Oxford University Press, 1993.
36. Graham JR, Watts D, Timbrook RE: Detecting fake-good and fake-bad MMPI-2 profiles. J Personality Assess 57:264–277, 1991.
37. Greene RL: Assessment of malingering and defensiveness by objective personality measures. In Rogers R (ed): Clinical Assessment of Malingering and Deception, 2nd ed. New York, Guilford Press, 1997, pp 169–207.
38. Greene RL: The MMPI-2/MMPI: An interpretive manual. Boston, Allyn & Bacon, 1991.
39. Guilmette TJ, Hart KJ, Guilianao AJO: Malingering detection: The use of a force-choice method in identifying organic versus simulated memory impairment. Clin Neuropsychol 7:59–69, 1993.
40. Heaton RK, Smith HH, Lehman RAW, Vogt AT: Prospects for faking believable deficits on neuropsychological testing. J Consult Clin Psychol 46:892–900, 1978.
41. Hildreth DH, Breidenbach WC, Lister GD, Hodges AD: Detection of submaximal effort by use of the rapid exchange grip. J Hand Surg 14a 4:742–745, 1989.
42. Koss MP, Butcher JN: A comparison of patients' self-report with other sources of clinical information. J Research Personality 7:225–236, 1973.
43. Kropp PR, Rogers R: Understanding malingering: Motivation, method and detection. In Lewis M, Saarni C (eds): Lying and Deception in Everday Life. New York, Guilford Press, 1993.
44. Lipowski ZJ: Somatization: The concept and its clinical application. Am J Psychiatry 145:1358–1368, 1988.
45. Main CJ, Waddell G: Spine update: Behavioral responses to examination, a reappraisal of the interpretation of "nonorganic signs." Spine 23:2367–2371, 1998.
46. Matheson LN: Symptom magnification syndrome: part I: description and definition. Ind Rehabil 4(1), 1991.
47. Mechanic D: The concept of illness behavior. J Chronic Disability 15:189–194, 1961.
48. Overholser JC: Differential diagnosis of malingering and factitious disorder with physical symptoms. Behav Sci Law 8:55–65, 1990.
49. Pankratz L: Procedures for the assessment and treatment of functional sensory deficits. J Consult Clin Psychol 47:409–410, 1979.
50. Pankratz L: A new technique for the assessment and modification of feigned memory deficit. Perceptual and Motor Skills 57:367–372, 1983.
51. Pankratz L, Binder LM, Wilcox L: Assessment of an exaggerated somatosensory deficit with symptom validity assessment [Letter]. Arch Neurol 4:798, 1987.
52. Pankratz L, Fausti S, Peed S: A forced-choice technique to evaluate deafness in the hysterical or malingering patient. J Consult Clin Psychol 43:421–422, 1975.
53. Pilowsky I: The concept of abnormal illness behavior. Psychosomatics 31:207–214, 1990.
54. Rogers R: Towards an empirical model of malingering and deception. Behav Sci Law 2:93–112, 1984.

55. Rogers R: The assessment of malingering within a forensic context. In Weisstub DN (ed): Law and Psychiatry: International Perspectives. Vol 3. New York, Plenum, 1987, pp 209–237.
56. Rogers R: Development of new classificatory model of malingering. Bull Am Acad Psychiatry Law 18:323–333, 1990.
57. Rogers R: Malingering. Harvard Mental Health Letter 10(9):3–5, 1994.
58. Rogers R, Bagby RM, Vincent A: Factitious disorders with predominantly psychological signs and symptoms: A conundrum for forensic experts. J Psychiatry Law 22:91–106, 1994.
59. Rogers R, Dion KL, Lynett E: Diagnostic validity of antisocial personality disorder. Law Hum Behav 16:677–689, 1992.
60. Rogers R, Harrell EH and Liff CD: Feigning neuropsychological impairment: A critical review of methodological and clinical considerations. Clin Psychol Review 13:255–274, 1993.
61. Rogers R, Nussbaum D: Interpreting response styles of inconsistent MMPI profiles. Forensic Reports 4:361–366, 1991.
62. Rogers R, Sewell KW, Salekin RT: A meta-analysis of malingering on the MMPI-2. Assessment 1:227–237, 1994.
63. Rosenhan D: On being sane in insane places. Science 172:250–258, 1973.
64. Rothke SE, Friedman AF, Dahlstrom WG, et al: MMPI-2 normative data for the F-K index: Implications for clinical, neuropsychological, and forensic practice. Assessment 1:1–15, 1994.
65. Smith GR Jr, Monson RA, Ray DC: Psychiatric consultation in somatization disorder: A randomized controlled study. New Engl J Med 314:1407–1413, 1986.
66. Spiro HR: Chronic factitious illness: Munchausen's syndrome. Arch Gen Psychiatry 18:569–579, 1968.
67. Stokes HM: The seriously uninjured hand—weakness of grip. J Occup Med 25:9:683–684, 1983.
68. Trueblood W, Binder LM: Psychologists' accuracy in identifying neuropsychological test protocols of clinical malingerers. Paper presented at the National Academy of Neuropsychology. San Francisco, October 1995.
69. Voiss DV: Occupational injury: Fact, fantasy, or fraud? In Weintraub MI (ed): Malingering and Conversion Reactions. Neurologic Clinics. Philadelphia, WB Saunders, May 1995, 431–446.
70. Waddell G, Main CJ, Morris EW, et al: Chronic low-back pain, psychologic distress, and illness behavior. Spine 9:2:209–213, 1984.
71. Waddell G, McCulloch JA, Kummel EG, Venner RM: Nonorganic physical signs in low-back pain. Spine 5:117–125, 1980.
72. Wasyliw O, Cavanaugh J: Simulation of brain damage: Assessment and decision rules. Bull Am Acad Psychiatry Law 17:373–386, 1989.

GERALD M. ARONOFF, MD
JEFFREY B. FELDMAN, PhD
THOMAS S. CAMPION, PT

MANAGEMENT OF CHRONIC PAIN AND CONTROL OF LONG-TERM DISABILITY

From the Mid-Atlantic Center for
Pain Management
Charlotte, North Carolina

Reprint requests to:
Gerald M. Aronoff, MD
Mid-Atlantic Center for Pain
Management
1901 Randolph Road
Charlotte, NC 28234

Estimates of the total cost of pain disorders in the U.S. range over $100 billion annually.[1,2] Among industrial injuries, back injuries are the most expensive and are a common cause of disability in adults younger than 45. Approximately 1% of the population is considered totally and permanently disabled by chronic back problems.[3] Between 1971 and 1981, the number of people with disabling back problems increased 168%, whereas the population increased by 12.5%.[4] Aronoff[5,6] has termed this a "disability epidemic" and believes it has become a major public health problem in the United States and other countries where entitlement programs are viewed as appealing alternatives to gainful employment. Compounding this epidemic are some medical practitioners who fail to distinguish between impairment and disability, as well as confusion concerning what constitutes maximum medical improvement (MMI). In a recent article, Aronoff and Feldman[7] have argued that confusion is further generated by the fact that chronic pain syndrome requires a biopsychosocial-economic perspective to evaluate and treat, while disability evaluation systems encourage rating of impairment using a biomedical perspective.

This article reviews the constellation of interacting symptoms which define chronic pain syndrome. Psychological and socioeconomic "red flags" for a poor return-to-work prognosis are delineated. The critical importance of physician statements to patients concerning their medical condition, resulting restrictions, and limitations is emphasized. The role of functional capacity evaluations in this process is discussed, with suggestions for their interpretation and use. The relationship between motivation, performance, and patients' beliefs about what they can do (self-efficacy) and what will happen when they return to work is reviewed. It is argued that this sense of self efficacy, often shaped by physician statements, as well as patient beliefs about return to work are of primary value in predicting successful rehabilitation.

CHRONIC PAIN SYNDROME AND DISABILITY

In discussing chronic pain, we are referring to chronic non-malignant pain as opposed to pain associated with cancer. The distinction between patients experiencing chronic pain and those exhibiting chronic pain syndrome (CPS) is largely made on the basis of behavior and functioning. CPS is not a diagnosis, but rather is a term to describe individuals who exhibit not only persistent pain, but also marked restriction in functional activities, life disruption, and dysfunctional pain behavior. **Pain behavior** is a form of abnormal illness behavior and includes audible and body language displays such as grimacing, bracing or guarding, persistent complaints, repeated visits to physicians and emergency rooms, and excessive use of analgesics and/or sedative drugs.[8,9] CPS is further characterized by symptoms of depression, anxiety, insomnia, physical deconditioning, chronic myalgias, family discord, and financial distress. Central to CPS and concurrent with these disability behaviors is a **disability conviction.** This is a belief that, because of chronic pain, one is unable to meet only occupational demands, but also domestic, family, and social responsibilities, and is unable to engage in avocational and recreational activities.

Matheson[10] presented a model suggesting that disability lies at the interface between functional limitations and role demands. Aronoff has emphasized that, "It is very important to evaluate motivation, which the AMA guides note cannot be ignored as a connecting link between impairment and disability."[11] Expanding upon these contributions, two of the current authors proposed a "cognitive-systems" model to clarify the relationship between chronic pain, and disability.[12] This cognitive-systems perspective recognizes the reciprocal relationship between patients' beliefs about their pain and the external systems by which they are influenced and that they in turn influence. Patients' beliefs about their pain and to what degree it affects their capabilities (functional self-efficacy) were found to be the strongest predictors of task performance (lifting)[13] and long-term rehabilitation.[14] These beliefs about pain can be affected by physician or attorney warnings; advice from family members; prior life history of injury, trauma, or abuse; personal values; and other personality factors. This sense of self-efficacy interacts with perceived demands of the job, physical, occupational, and psychosocial factors which can create adversarial relationships and/or disincentives to return to work. The development of CPS and its accompanying disability conviction therefore involves complex interactions among individuals in pain and the many people and systems that influence and inform their beliefs. Building upon Matheson's model, it can be stated that in the case of CPS, disability lies at the interface of numerous interacting systems which shape individuals' beliefs about their condition, what they can do, and what is in their best long-term interest.

Psychological Warning Signs

Highly relevant to chronic pain and disability are the interacting systems that comprise the individual's psychological constitution. A study by Gatchel et al.[15] clarified both the prevalence of psychological distress in chronic low back pain and the difficulty of using any one psychological diagnosis or factor as a prognostic indicator. They found that more than 90% of 152 disabled patients with low back pain entering an intensive 3-week functional restoration program obtained at least one Axis I diagnosis, and more than 50% obtained at least one Axis II diagnosis. Axis I diagnoses most commonly involved depression or anxiety, while Axis II diagnoses reflected a range of personality disorders. Interestingly, neither type nor degree of psychopathology were significantly predictive of a patient's ability to successfully return to work. This indicates that psychological factors create a high potential for disability following injury, but can be productively addressed through appropriate treatment in the form of comprehensive pain rehabilitation and/or functional restoration treatment programs that incorporate cognitive-behavioral treatment into a physical rehabilitation approach. It is for this reason, as we will later more fully elaborate, that patients with CPS should not be rated at MMI until they have received or refused such treatment or have been deemed inappropriate for such treatment. It is also most likely the case that Gatchel et al. did not find a specific diagnosis as statistically predictive of return to work for their sample because such an outcome is a product of numerous interacting psychological, physical, occupational, and socioeconomic factors. In a large sample, any one factor may not yield statistical significance while being clinically highly significant for an individual patient. We will first review some of the most common psychological "red flags" (Table 1) and then socioeconomic ones.

DEVELOPMENTAL HISTORY

Investigation of the developmental history of chronic pain patients is important because studies repeatedly indicate a high incidence of prior physical and/or sexual trauma in individuals suffering from CPS.[16-23] The subjective complaints of these pain patients seem grossly disproportionate to objective findings: patients frequently are unresponsive to traditional medical, pharmacological, or surgical approaches.[24] Brain imaging studies suggest limbic-system abnormalities in previously traumatized

TABLE 1.   Psychological "Red Flags"

Developmental history
    History of physical or sexual abuse
    Caretaker for younger siblings
    History of recurrent medical treatment for a variety of injuries/illnesses
    Family history of disability
    History of multiple unstable relationships
    History of psychological problems
Behavioral
    High degree of pain behavior and/or functional impairment
    Doctor shopping or excessive use of healthcare services
    Drug-seeking behavior/substance abuse
    Poor compliance
Affective
    High degree of depression, anger, emotional lability
    Indifference/lack of distress
Cognitive
    Disability conviction
    Belief that there should be a medical cure
    Fear of reinjury or condition worsening
    Belief that one cannot return to work or will not be rehired
    Perceived adequacy of treatment
Current family
    Family functions not being carried out
    Reinforcement of disability by family members
    Other family members on disability
    Marital conflict/dissatisfaction/instability

individuals.[40] Animal studies demonstrate that high-level amygdala stimulation interferes with hippocampal functioning.[25] In humans, hippocampal dysfunction results in impairment of declarative or verbal memory.[26] Memories may very well be encoded emotionally by the amygdala, with individuals unable to place them into a meaningful context. This would correspond to the wordless fear and panic triggered in patients with post-traumatic stress disorder (PTSD) by a relevant stimulus. Decreased hippocampal functioning further causes hyperresponsiveness to stimuli, most likely by causing incoming stimuli to be interpreted in the direction of "emergency" (fight or flight) responses. This appears consistent with decreased serotonin activity and elevated catecholamine levels found in PTSD patients.[25]

The reactivation of a fear/emergency reaction in PTSD patients by stimuli associated with trauma may be viewed as a process of **state-dependent learning.**[27] Pain may trigger similar responses from individuals who have suffered painful traumatic events. In other words, pain may trigger subcortically mediated emotional responses that escape cortical and possibly hippocampal inhibitory control. The association between CPS and PTSD might explain the high degree of anxiety, emotional reactivity, and hyperalgesia in many chronic pain patients. Responses which seem grossly disproportionate to observed peripheral injury or damage may make sense given such conditioned central reactivity. Similarly, symptoms of depression and the responsiveness of both chronic pain patients and PTSD patients of serotonergic agents may be due to common neurobiological processes. The automatic unconscious triggering of responses to pain is congruent with Melzack's concept of neuromodules.[28,29] Extrapolating from his work with phantom limb pain, Melzack argues that the brain generates the pain experience, and can do so in the absence of peripheral input. Melzack postulates that pain is processed as "neuromodules" or networks which include linkages between virtually every region of the brain. This would certainly include linkages to the limbic system, with such activation causing a threshold to be reached which would activate a neuromodule, at times with minimal peripheral input.

The association between a developmental history significant for much stress, trauma, and unmet dependency needs has long been noted in the psychiatric and medical literature and explained in psychodynamic terms as causing a **pain-prone personality.**[30,31] Often due to parental dysfunction, or simply due to family size, such individuals while still children themselves had to take care of younger siblings and at times their parents. Aronoff[32] has indicated that chronic pain provides an opportunity for such individuals to get early unmet dependency needs satisfied. Their dysfunctional stance is their way of saying, "Now it is my turn to be taken care of." In somatic terms they are saying "my life hurts," yet all too frequently their physical complaint is treated with a conventional medical remedy.

These individuals may have learned how to satisfy their emotional needs through physical symptoms. For such patients, early parenting may have treated medical complaints—but not emotional symptoms—as deserving of attention. Patients may therefore have learned that the way to get attention, nurturance, and care is to complain about physical symptoms. For a more in-depth discussion of the wide range of somatoform disorders in which patients can express their emotional distress through physical symptoms, the reader is referred to a recent article on preventing iatrogenic disability.[7]

Alternatively, patients may have learned through parents, other family members, or other role models that disability is a socially acceptable way to live. A family history of disability should alert physicians that such patients may simply be carrying out what they have learned to be the family destiny and may be aligning themselves with family members for whom closeness in more functional ways is problematic.

Finally, in terms of development, a history of psychological problems and/or unstable relationships may be an ominous warning sign. The field of behavioral medicine has taught us that psychosocial stressors cause or exacerbate multiple physical symptoms, including those with underlying medical pathophysiology.[7] A life history of emotional and interpersonal turmoil and dysfunctional relationships can predispose an individual to psychophysiological conditions.

BEHAVIORAL FACTORS

Emotional distress can be displayed through many pain behaviors (Table 2). As noted by Turk & Okifuji,[33] "It is important that pain behaviors not be considered a lack of motivation for getting well or malingering." They clarify that there is no conscious deception on the patient's part, but rather unintended performance of pain behaviors resulting from reinforcement contingencies. In other words, it is learned behavior of which the patient is unaware. Waddel agrees that pain behavior (including what has come to be termed "Waddel signs") is nonvolitional. He notes that:

From a clinical perspective, the behavioral symptoms and signs can be considered as a form of communication between patient and doctor . . . More, they may be regarded as an overt clinical expression of the patient's distress about the severity of the problem.[8]

More recently, Waddel has argued that:

Illness behavior does not just happen, it is learned. It is not fixed, but is a dynamic process over time, and health care may play a key role in its development. . . .Clinical observation of illness behavior is clearly only one facet of a complex phenomenon. We must assess the whole clinical picture before we can begin to understand illness behavior.[9]

Physicians who negatively react to such behavior, viewing the patient as a "nut," will most likely only amplify the patient's pain behavior as he or she non-verbally attempts to communicate, "But I really do hurt, I know there's something wrong." Furthermore, it is important to note that such pain behavior need not be indicative of a poor prognosis. Hazard, Bendix, and Fenwick[34] found that pain behavior, termed by them "disability exaggeration," did not predict treatment outcome. Examining change scores, however, Werneke, Harris and Lechter[35] found that "behavioral signs" significantly decreased for those who returned to work, but not for those who did not. It appears, therefore, that the reduction in psychological distress (exhibited as pain behavior) in the course of treatment—rather than the degree of distress upon initial evaluation—is the salient factor in predicting return to work.

Feeling disbelieved or discounted, patients often go from one physician to the next looking for the one who "will really listen and understand my pain." Pain syndrome patients, in their desperate search for the elusive cure, often "chase windmills" and convince their doctors to perform a myriad of invasive tests and procedures.

TABLE 2.   Pain Behavior

Vocal complaints—verbal
Vocal complaints—nonverbal (moans, groans, gasps)
Down-time because of pain greater than 60 min/day
Facial grimaces
Standing posture distorted
Mobility—walking labored or with marked limp
Body language—clutching, rubbing site of pain
Use of visible physical supports—corset, cane, crutches
Stationary movement—frequent movement or shifts of position
Medication—frequent demands for increased dose, frequency, or stronger narcotics

As a result of their pain behaviors, many experience iatrogenic complications, suffering, and disability. Those involved in their treatment must find improved ways to detect this highly susceptible population, establish a therapeutic alliance, and short-circuit their pain careers. Our health care system of finite resources cannot rely solely on the traditional methods of medical and surgical approaches so often used with this population.[36] Requests for medication may represent an attempt to get relief of pain and suffering. Alternately, such drug-seeking behavior may reflect a substance abuse problem in which the pain becomes a more socially accepted way of asking for drugs. Poor compliance with treatment, with the patient going from one physician to the next, or quick requests for a change in medications before following the recommended regimen may indicate a substance abuse problem or that the pain meets certain psychological needs, and wellness is a threat.

Pain behavior that more pervasively affects an individual's life through an inordinate degree of functional limitation has been termed **abnormal illness behavior.** In an effort to quantify such behavior Main and Waddel[37] developed the Illness Behavior Questionnaire. However, the psychometric properties of the instrument have been questioned,[33] and the instruments most commonly used to measure dysfunction due to pain are the Roland and Morris Disability Questionnaire[38] and the Oswestry Disability Scale.[39] In our clinic we have found that the mean score among patients presenting with CPS is 18 of the 24 Roland and Morris items. Roberts[40] found the Roland questionnaire simpler, faster, and more acceptable to patients than the Oswestry, agreeing with Deyo[41] that it provides a more sensitive measure of early and acute disability. Waddel believes the Roland gives the best measure of recovery or the early development of chronic pain and disability, viewing it as the best available tool at present for most clinical use or research.[9] While we also use the Roland, the benefit of the Oswestry is that scores are categorized in the mild, moderate, severe, or bedridden range of disability. We find it helpful to point out to patients who have come daily to the clinic 8 hours a day, for up to 4 weeks, that their reported degree of pain-related disability places them within the "bedridden" range on the Oswestry.

AFFECTIVE FACTORS

Chronic pain patients often present with significant, anger, depression, and/or emotional lability. Among these, depression has been most widely noted, generating considerable discussion in the field. Gallagher[42,43] and Romano and Turner[44] found a wide variability among studies of concurrent depression in patients with pain (10–78%) and pain in patients with depression (27–100%). Atkinson[45] noted that up to 50% of patients with chronic pain may suffer a major depressive episode at some point in their pain syndrome. Lindsay and Wycoff[46] noted that 87% of patients referred to a pain center were depressed, with 83% of these showing improvement in their pain when treated with antidepressants. Magni[47] found in a prospective study of 607 workers in three metal industry plants that depressive symptoms predicted musculoskeletal disorders. A significant problem with many studies relating pain and depression is the lack of controls for physical and medication factors that confounded the diagnosis of major depression.[48] Numerous studies suggest that depression can be both a significant causative factor and a common result of chronic pain.

The most frequently used self-report measure of depression is the Beck Depression Inventory.[49] It is a self-report measure composed of 21 items that can be completed in 5 minutes. Score results are categorized from indicating no affective distress, to a mild mood disorder, to mild, to moderate, and severe depression. While high scores need to be taken seriously, especially if suicidal ideation or plans are acknowledged, scores in the mild to moderate range may overestimate the degree of depression in chronic pain patients due to overlap between pain-related physiological symptoms and affect disorder symptoms.[50]

In our experience, a red flag of greater concern than a report of mild to moderate depression is a *lack* of emotional distress expressed on the Beck and/or in interview. Individuals acknowledging depression usually are stating that they are unhappy with their current life situation, and therefore have motivation for change. They have greater rehabilitation potential than individuals who exhibit "la belle indifference," not seeming distressed by their pain and limitations in functioning. We believe these individuals are content being disabled.

COGNITIVE FACTORS

Patients' belief about their pain, its cause, how they should be treated for it, and their ability to function are critical factors in the generation of disability. Jensen et al. found that beliefs about pain were better predictors of post-treatment functioning than following prescribed behaviors such as walking and exercise regimes. Similarly, Reitsma and Miejlin[51] found that the best predictor of continued medical utilization and dysfunction among individuals with chronic pain was the ongoing belief that there must be a cure for their pain. The most thoroughly researched instrument for assessing relevant beliefs about pain is the **Survey of Pain Attitudes** (SOPA) developed by Jensen and associates.[52] In a subsequent paper,[12] the current authors delineated corresponding beliefs among family members which would reinforce such beliefs. These dysfunctional beliefs largely revolve around notions that hurt means harm, that rest and inactivity are the appropriate responses to chronic pain, and family members should not expect the person in pain to do much. Furthermore, the belief that there must be a cure for the pain leads the patient and the family to believe that they have not as yet received adequate treatment, and they continue to search for "the right doctor" who can "fix what's wrong." Other beliefs, not on the SOPA but critical to issues of return to work, involve patients' beliefs about whether they can or should have to return to some kind of work, and more specifically, whether they can return to their previous job. Interacting with this is the commonly expressed view that once employees are injured and file worker's compensation claims, the company will find a reason to terminate them.[3] Thus, the worker views attempts to return to work as unwise.

CURRENT FAMILY CHARACTERISTICS

The family environment is the primary one in which appropriate adaptation or maladaptation can occur, and families can be either the physicians' best allies or their worst saboteurs.[12] A **cognitive-systems perspective** was proposed to assess the affect of chronic pain on the patient and family by evaluating the degree to which family functions are carried out and by whom, the cognitive beliefs of the patient and family members that support functioning or dysfunction, and the interaction patterns between family members. Often most evident is the fact that vocational functioning is omitted or curtailed, with significant financial damage to the family. Less immediately, spiritual, social, recreational, and sexual activities are disrupted, as is emotional support. Other family members, typically the spouse, may take on the patient's responsibilities. In this way and/or by providing a great deal of attention to the person in pain, caring family members may reinforce disability. Alternately, a family member (or members) already disabled may influence the patient to join them in disability, with it becoming an accepted family role. Finally, pain can either generate a great deal of marital dissatisfaction and conflict, or serve as a means of masking such instability. Spouses may avoid dealing with problematic issues, believing, for instance, that the patient should not be troubled when in pain and needy.

Socioeconomic Warning Signs

The literature on work-related injury and return to work is characterized by inconsistency in subject samples, variables assessed, process, and outcome measures. Patient groups vary in selection criteria, nature of injury, type of work, pain duration, disability levels, and multiple socioeconomic and vocational variables. Outcome measures vary in measures of pain, function, disability, work status, and duration of follow-up.[6,51] Nevertheless, the clearest trend in this flawed literature is that psychosocial factors are more important determinants of return to work than physical factors.[54] Lancourt and Kettelhut,[55] in a prospective study of 134 patients with lower back pain, found that patients who returned to work had fewer job, personal, or family-related problems. There were no significant differences between patients who returned to work and those who did not when comparing myelograms, CT scans, or x-rays. Gallagher et al.[47] similarly found psychosocial factors to be more important determinants of return to work than physical factors, and pointed out the need to adjust for the confounding effects of age and length of time out of work in assessing any variables. Tate[56] evaluated data from 200 worker's compensation cases, finding workers' age, education, wages before injury, and job seniority as predictive of return to work. In contrast to the prior studies cited, Tate found that severity of the injury *was* a significant predictor of return to work, with back impairment a particular risk factor.

Probably the best known research concerning industrial back injury is that of Bigos and associates,[57,58] who prospectively studied 3020 aircraft employees at the Boeing Company for reports of back problems. A history of prior medical treatment for a back problem was the only physical variable predictive of reporting acute back pain at work. The most predictive individual factors were job task dissatisfaction as measured by a modified work APGAR scale, and distress as reported on scale 3 of the Minnesota Multiphasic Personality Inventory. Note that the three factors in the study cited above (job satisfaction, psychological distress, and prior back injury) only improved prediction of back injury reports by 7–8.6%.[20] Furthermore, in contrast to the most popularized finding of the Boeing study, Feyer et al.[59] did not find work dissatisfaction to be related to low back pain disability.

What emerges from this body of research is that no single physical, psychological, or vocational factor, nor group of factors, consistently predicts injury or successful rehabilitation.[60] Rather, these phenomena reflect multi-factor, multi-system interactions between physical, occupational, developmental, social, interpersonal, psychological, and economic variables.

OCCUPATIONAL FACTORS

Despite Feyer et al.[61] finding a lack of relationship between job satisfaction and return to work, it has been our clinical experience, in accord with Bigos et al.,[62,63] that injured workers who are unhappy at work are less likely to return to their jobs. Reports of conflict with co-workers and/or the patient's supervisor are poor prognostic signs, as are poor performance evaluations or disciplinary actions. These and other factors such as boredom, monotony, or feeling underutilized may indicate a low degree of job satisfaction. A recent change in position or job demands may indicate that patients feel as if they have been demoted, or conversely put them in a position where they feel overwhelmed. A work history of multiple short-term jobs may indicate social or adjustment difficulties, antisocial behavior, or simply a poor work ethic. Correspondingly, a brief period on the job prior to injury tends to be a poor prognostic sign. Recent or rumored plant closings or layoffs tend to discourage return to work, with the patient reasonably believing that there will not be a job to return to for long; disability appears to be a better alternative than unemployment. Similarly, work shifts longer than 8 hours negatively impact the patient's sense of confidence in being able to successfully return to work (RTW).

Other factors that affect successful return to work are the age of the employee (with extreme youth as well as age having reduced probability of RTW), education level, and transferable skills. Similarly, the level of pre-injury wages and amount of wage replacement when out of work are significant factors.

Highly significant is the finding in a number of studies that there is a dramatic decrease in the probability of return to work the longer the patient is out of work. By the time an individual with an industrial injury is out of work 6 months, there is only a 50% probability of return to work. At two years, the probability is minimal.[9] In their review of the literature on preventing disability from work-related low-back pain, Frank and colleagues[64] point to the need for timely and appropriate intervention. Citing the Agency for Healthcare Policy and Research (AHCPR) guidelines, they point out that most clinical interventions in the acute stage (up to 3 weeks post-injury) appear to be ineffective, at times generating iatrogenic illness. In contrast, intervention seems essential in the subacute phase (3–12 weeks) to prevent CPS and long-term disability. Frank and colleagues emphasize that an essential element of success of subacute-stage intervention in returning people to work is to involve the workplace explicitly in the process. A supportive workplace response to injury needs to start when the pain is first reported. An individualized, nonadversarial approach which includes early return to work should follow promptly, to circumvent the development of disability behavior. This is in contrast to the "adversarial care"[3] which all too often develops in the management of industrial injury patients.

Bigos et al., citing the work of Guest and Drummond,[65] have most thoroughly and persuasively argued that this system is inherently harmful to individuals trapped within it:

> The creation of the term industrial back pain apparently fostered the development of adversarial attitudes and expensive systems that have only worsened the burden by expanding costs without returning the injured worker to productivity. "Adversarial help" seems, and mostly is, a contradiction in terms. In any event, this "adversarial help" system, although a growing expense, has had little effect in aiding the worker or society by reaching the goal of keeping our populous productive until retirement age.

Contributing to this adversarial situation is what many workers describe as an unwritten rule that the likelihood of job loss is markedly increased following an injury claim.[3] Patients will usually not recover from an injury without a perception of a viable alternative to disability.

Some patients feel it necessary to have an attorney advocate for them in this adversarial system. The degree to which this represents a red flag is a matter of some controversy. Cummings[66] has claimed that 90% of attorneys drop the case if the person wants to return to work. Similarly, Mundy, Moore, Corey, and Mundy[62] report attorneys discouraging early return to work or modified duty. In their review of the literature, Gallagher, Williams, and Skelly argued that evidence from prior studies concerning these factors is inconclusive. In their empirical study, Gallagher and colleagues found that, "neither compensation status nor involvement of a lawyer significantly improved prediction of employment status 6 months later."[47] In our clinical experience, patients retaining attorneys soon after injury have delayed recovery significantly more than those who get an attorney only after what they perceive to be an extended period of not getting adequate care or being treated unfairly. Probably most important concerning whether attorney involvement should be viewed as a red flag is whether the attorney advises the patient to seek disability rather than return to work.

Finally, and probably of greatest relevance, is the **advice of the physician.** Catchlove and Cohen[67] demonstrated a significantly better return-to-work rate when patients were directed to do so either during or after treatment, compared with a control group for whom return to work was not emphasized. Hall and associates[68] in a more recent study similarly demonstrated that a recommendation to return to work without restrictions facilitated successful outcome. In contrast, a restriction intended to return a patient to a reduced level of job demand decreased the likelihood of the patient successfully working at a 4-month follow-up. Catchlove and Cohen argued that patients view themselves as incapable of full recovery if return to work is not encouraged. Hall and colleagues expanded upon this, stating that, "An unwarranted restriction implies disability and may become a self-fulfilling prophecy."[69] They note that since research indicates no correlation between subjective pain ratings and the patient's ability to accomplish physical activities, the patient's subjective complaints should not be the basis for determination of restrictions or disability.

Aronoff has stated: "One should not underestimate the importance of physicians' authoritarian guidance, which can be offered as supportive paternalism. Patients will either live up to our expectations that they need not be disabled or, conversely, become invalids unnecessarily through learned helplessness. It is our ethical responsibility to improve patients' health whenever possible. Their physical, emotional, social, and spiritual well-being is more likely to be realized with the self-esteem that results from feeling useful from gainful employment rather than from disability."

If return to work recommendations should be made on the basis of objective information and not on a subjective report of pain, what objective measures should be used? In their search for objective information many practitioners use the results of functional capacity evaluations.

FUNCTIONAL CAPACITY EVALUATIONS

Functional capacity evaluations (FCEs) may be viewed as a link between healthcare providers and industry, as well as an opportunity for individuals to move from viewing themselves as recovering patients to seeing themselves as productive workers.[71] One of the difficult aspects of treating worker's compensation patients is determining what activities a worker can safely perform. The number of hours worked per day, safe lifting amounts, positional tolerances, and other activities of a worker's daily functioning need to be determined. Choosing a method for obtaining these parameters is a matter of debate. It is generally felt that getting this information through a functional approach is the most accurate.[67] Before the development of FCEs, the determination of an injured worker's return-to-work status was based on an impairment rating, the diagnosis, and simply asking the patient what he or she could do. Physicians generally would briefly interview and observe patients, who usually were not asked to do any work-related activity. The physician was forced to make an educated guess and fill out the physical functioning form requested by the employer and/or insurance company. There was no scientific basis to the way in which functional capacities were estimated. Due to the limited amount of patient information available, and the physician having to largely rely on past experience and clinical intuition, this system often resulted in return-to-work parameters that were very conservative and prevented the injured worker from returning to full employment. Often the employer would be unable to offer employment within the low work restrictions.[72] This system was obviously inefficient, since due to limited information the physician typically waited longer than necessary to decide on the patient's work level.

FCEs have evolved in an attempt to provide physicians with objective information regarding a patient's safe functional ability. They generally offer significant advantages to the diagnostic/impairment rating system. They have become an integral part of work injury prevention and rehabilitation. They define a person's safe, functional ability to perform work, and whether these abilities match the job requirements.[73] The Occupational Safety and Health Administration (OSHA) promotes the use of FCEs in an effort to provide a safe return to work for injured clients, and the Americans With Disabilities Act (ADA) emphasizes identifying an individual's ability for work, as well as any accommodations that may be necessary.[74] FCEs have also become an important piece of documentation in legal proceedings concerning a client's ability to earn wages.[75] In short, the FCE has become a widely accepted tool for determining work readiness, for making disability determinations, for setting rehab treatment goals and plans of care, and for closing cases.[69]

Currently, there are a number of FCEs available commercially.[76] In addition, many clinics have developed their own versions. These FCEs vary in how they assess sincerity of effort, use isometric testing, use generic versus job-specific testing, and their methods of projecting endurance for an 8-hour day. There also are wide variations in the level of training and experience of clinicians administering the test.[69] FCEs vary in how well they are able to reliably, objectively, safely, and accurately predict a client's ability to perform work. Due to the increased role of the FCE in helping insurers, physicians, and employers make decisions. FCEs need to meet credibility requirements. It is important that the referral source know what they are getting in the FCE. The following is a brief overview of what comprises a sound FCE.[67]

An FCE needs to provide information about the 20 physical demands of work described by the Department of Labor in the *Dictionary of Occupational Titles*. In addition, the intensity and frequency of work tolerance is described, and the level of work the client is capable of performing is classified as sedentary, light, medium, heavy, or very heavy. Position tolerances are also rated according to whether a client can perform them constantly, frequently, occasionally, and never. If a job description is available that is detailed enough, then it can be used to provide a match between the client's abilities and the job demands. In short, the FCE should be **comprehensive.**[67]

The FCE should also provide **objective** and **standardized** means to measure a client's performance. Each task of the FCE needs to be administered and scored in a systematic way. This is essential if the FCE is to be repeatable and an accurate predictor of the client's capacity for work. The FCE must be as free from observer bias as possible, and this must be demonstrated through reliability and validity studies.[67]

An FCE's **reliability** refers to how consistent the results of the testing are from one examiner to another, and from one administration of the test to another: interrater reliability and test-retest reliability. Without this, one cannot know if the information is accurate and if it is a fair representation of a client's abilities.[67]

An FCE's **validity** is essentially a measure of how predictable the FCE is regarding the client's functioning in the "real world." In other words, if an FCE indicates that a person is safe to return to work at a particular job, does that actually happen? How long does the client stay at this job? Is he or she able to tolerate the job for 8 hours per day/40 hours per week? How often does the client get reinjured, or quit? It is important to note that the test validity is *not* a measure of the client's sincerity of effort; *test validity is established through research* and is not dependent upon client cooperation. If the client self-limits, then the test is a measure of what the client was willing to do, and is still predictive of what they most likely will be willing to do in the workplace. In that sense the test remains valid.[67]

The reliability and validity of these physical performance tests are crucial to their success in the real world. If a test is not reliable, then a client could be sent to a different therapist and get a completely different result. If the test is not valid, then no one would know whether the information is accurate. As medical care practitioners we have an ethical obligation to provide reliable and valid assessments, particularly if the results influence litigation.

FCEs are also requested to provide information regarding the client's **sincerity of effort.** Many different means have been tried in an attempt to do this, including obtaining co-efficient of variation scores, using Waddell's nonorganic signs, and using the bell-shaped curve with isometric grip strength testing. No current research supports any of these methods for determining sincerity of effort. At best, what we can do is document whether a client is performing to a maximum level by comparing their physical signs of effort with their willingness to perform. If the client limits him or herself prior to exhibiting maximum effort, this can, of course, be documented. The *reason(s)* underlying this behavior, whether fear or reinjury, pain, misunderstanding of the instructions, or an intentional attempt to manipulate the test, cannot be determined during the FCE. Nevertheless, a well constructed and administered FCE remains a good predictor of the client's work level, since it is unlikely that he/she will be any more willing to perform at work than they are for the therapist during the FCE.[77]

During the FCE, the clinician must be careful to not cause further injury to the client. This can occur by stressing the client beyond the point where their activities are unsafe. Close observation of the client's movements and an ability to recognize unsafe movements are crucial in knowing when to stop the client on a particular task, as well as in knowing when the client has stopped before reaching safe maximum effort. This is one reason why it is important that the clinician administering the test have a certain level of training to ensure safety, quality, and consistency.[68]

After the FCE has been completed, the results are summarized in a report and sent to the referral source for interpretation. FCEs often generate restrictions in what a worker can do, whether in the amount of frequency of lifting or carrying, in positional tolerances, or in the client's endurance to manage an 8-hour work day. Generally, the goal is that the restrictions match whatever job was held before the injury. This is especially true with those clients who have recently completed a rehabilitation program and are being released to return to work.[67] A recently published study from the Canadian Back Institute (CBI) looked at the effect of discharge recommendations on the outcome of clients who were returned to work without restrictions. The clients who were returned to work without restrictions had a higher success rate than those who returned to work with restrictions—84% compared to 47%. The CBI stated that, "The probability of failure increases significantly with . . . restrictions.[64] For those clients who have recently completed an FCE, if their current abilities allow them to do their job without restrictions, *they need to know they can return to this particular job without restrictions.*

There continues to be confusion for end-users (physicians, employers, rehab personnel) primarily in the interpretation of FCEs. For example, FCEs are often used in helping to determine what a client's functional abilities are once they have reached maximum medical improvement (MMI). It is important to remember that the FCE is a **snapshot in time** of that person's abilities, and that with additional time and continued use of good body mechanics and posture, as well as a regular exercise program, the client's functional abilities may improve. This describes a difference then between a person at MMI and what might be called their maximum *functional* improvement.

Hopefully, the above information will be helpful to those who use FCEs to make decisions regarding a client's work or disability status. The goal of the FCE is to provide the referral source with information about the client that is clear, unbiased, reliable, and valid.

CONCLUSION:

As stated by Fordyce: "People are complex. Their pain problems are complex. They—patient and clinician—exist in a complex world." Aronoff, citing the AMA guides, has previously emphasized that it is very important to evaluate motivation, which cannot be ignored as a connecting link between impairment and disability. We can view it as axiomatic that people are motivated to act according to what they understand to be in their best interest. We have reviewed in this paper many of the factors or red flags that might lead patients to believe that it is not in their best interest to return to work following an injury. No single factor nor combination of factors is universally predictive of functional disability nor return to work. Accumulating evidence suggests for up to four weeks post-injury that medical intervention other than conservative care is rarely indicated unless there are specific factors suggestive of organic pathology. Critical to preventing disability is intervention in the subacute phase, 3–12 weeks post injury. It is at the 3–4 week point that the red flags noted in this paper need to be assessed and addressed.

Treatment is most successful in the context of a functionally oriented return-to-work program that involves the employer and provides training in coping skills and pain management techniques. Once patients develop CPS, a more comprehensive interdisciplinary pain rehabilitation program geared towards functional restoration is often necessary. A cognitive-behavioral approach can assist with resolving cognitive distortions, dysfunctional pain behaviors, and disability convictions in a supportive and therapeutic milieu which enables the patient to believe that return to work is not only possible, but desirable.

Furthermore, while temporary restrictions that enable the worker to return to modified duty and avoid being taken out of work appear advised in the acute and subacute phases, long-term restrictions are contraindicated for successful recovery and

---

TABLE 3   Socioeconomic "Red Flags"

Occupational
    Conflict with co-workers and/or supervisor
    Recent or repeated disciplinary action
    Poor performance evaluations
    Low job satisfaction
    Recent change in position or job demands
    Multiple short-term jobs
    Brief period on the job prior to injury
    Recent or rumored plant closings or layoffs
    No light duty or modified positions
    Greater than 8 hour shifts
Time out of work
Wage replacement
Age
Education and transferable skills
Adversarial relationship with insurance company,
    rehabilitation professionals, and/or employer
Attorney advice against return to work
Physician advice against return to work

---

return to work. Work-related injury and disability is not a biomedical, but a **biopsy-chosocial-economic problem.** As concluded by Frank and colleagues,[59] piecemeal approaches that address only one factor or only one phase of disability generally are not successful. Collaborative problem-solving that involves changes on the part of government, unions, employers, the insurance industry, and the legal and medical professions is necessary.

REFERENCES

1. Gallagher RM: Behavioral and biobehavioral treatment in chronic pain: Perspectives on the evidence of effectiveness. Mind/Body Medicine 1997;2:176–183.
2. Aronoff GM, Dupuy DN: Evaluation and management of back pain: Preventing disability. J Back Musculoskel Rehabil 1997;9:109–124.
3. Bigos SJ, Baker R, Lee S: A definition and approach to helping the patient with a return to work predicament. Phys Med Rehabil Clin North Am 1993;4:109–123.
4. Gatchel RJ, Polatin PB, Mayer TG, Garcy PD: Psychopathology and the rehabilitation of patients with chronic low back pain disability. Arch Phys Med Rehabil 1994;75:666–670.
5. Aronoff GM, McClary PW: Multidisciplinary treatment of intractable chronic pain syndromes. Adv Pain Res Ther 1990;13:270.
6. Aronoff GM: The disability epidemic. Clin J Pain 1989;5:203–204 (editorial).
7. Aronoff GM, Feldman JB: Preventing iatrogenic disability from chronic pain. Curr Review Pain 1993;3:67–77.
8. Waddell G, Pilowsky I, Bond M: Clinical assessment and interpretation of abnormal illness behavior in low back pain. Pain 1989;39:41–53.
9. Waddell G: The Back Pain Revolution. Edinburgh, Churchill Livingstone, 1998, pp 166–167.
10. Matheson LN: Functional capacity evaluation. In Demeter S, Anderson GE, Smith G (eds): Disability Evaluation. St. Louis, Mosby, pp 168–188.
11. Aronoff GM: Pain. In Demeter S, Andersson G, Smith G. (eds): Disability Evaluation. St. Louis, Mosby, 1996, pp 529–542.
12. Feldman JB, Phillips LM, Aronoff GM: A cognitive systems approach to treating chronic pain patients and their families. In Aronoff GM: Evaluation and Treatment of Chronic Pain, 3rd ed. Baltimore, Wiliams & Wilkins, 1998, pp 313–322.
13. Lackner J, Carosella A, Feuerstein M: Pain expectancies, pain, and functional self-efficacy expectancies as determinants of disability in patients with chronic low back disorders. J Consult Clin Psychol 1996;64:212–220.
14. Jensen MP, Turner JA, Romano JM: Correlates of improvement in multi-disciplinary treatment of chronic pain. J Consul Clin Psychol 1994;62:172–179.
15. Gatchel RJ, Polatin PB, Mayer TG, & Garcy PD. Psychopathology and the rehabilitation of patients with chronic low back pain disability. Archives of Physical Medicine and Rehabilitation 1994;75:666–670.
16. Grunau RVE, Whitfield ME, Petrie JH, Fryer EL: Early pain experience, child and family factors as precursors of somatization: a prospective study of extremely premature and full term children. Pain 1994;56:353–359.
17. Wurtele SK, Kaplan GM, Keaimes M: Childhood sexual abuse among chronic pain patients. Clin J Pain 1990;40:110–113.
18. Blair JA, Blair RS, Rueckert P: Pre-injury emotional trauma and chronic pain, an unexpected finding. Spine 1994;19:1146–1147.
19. Van der Kolk B, Pelcovitz D, Roth S, et al: Dissociation, somatization, and affect dysregulation: The complexity of adaptation of trauma. Am J Psychiatry 1996;153:83–93.
20. Schofferman J, Anderson D, Hines R, et al: Childhood psychological trauma and chronic refractory low-back pain. Clin J Pain 1993;9:260–265.
21. Blair JA, Blair RS, Rueckert P: Pre-injury emotional trauma and chronic pain, an unexpected finding. Spine 1994;19:1146–1147.
22. Van der Kolk B, Pelcovitz D, Roth S, et al: Dissociation, somatization, and affect dysregulation: The complexity of adaptation of trauma. Am J Psychiatry 1996;153:83–93.
23. Schofferman J, Anderson D, Hines R, et al: Childhood psychological trauma and chronic refractory low-back pain. Clin J Pain 1993;9:260–265.
24. Aronoff GM: Psychiatric aspects of nonmalignant chronic pain: A new nosology. Evaluation and Treatment of Chronic Pain, 3rd ed. Baltimore, Williams and Wilkins, 1998; pp 291–300.
25. van der Kolk B: The body keeps the score: Memory and the evolving psychobiology of posttraumatic stress. Harvard Rev Psychiatry 1994;1(5):253–265.
26. Le Doux JE: Emotion, memory and the brain. Scientific American June 1994; pp 50–57.
27. Rossi E: The Psychobiology of Mind-Body Healing. N.Y., Norton, 1986.

28. Melzack R: Phantom limbs. Scientific American 1992;266(4)120–6.
29. Melzack R: Pain and stress: A new perspective. In 89–106.
30 Engel GL: Psychogenic pain and the pain-prone patient. Am J Medicine 1959;26:899–918.
31. Blumer D, Heilbronn M: Chronic pain as a variant of depressive disease: The pain-prone disorder. J Nerv Ment Dis 1982;170:381–406.
32. Aronoff GM: Psychiatric aspects of nonmalignant chronic pain: A new nosology. Evaluation and Treatment of Chronic Pain, 3rd ed. Baltimore, Williams and Wilkins, 1998, pp 291–300.
33. Turk DC, Okifuji A: Evaluating the role of physical, operant, cognitive, and affective factors in pain behavior in chronic pain patients. Behav Mod 1997;259–280.
34. Hazard R, Haugh L, Reid S, Preble J, MacDonald L: Early prediction of chronic disability after occupational low back injury. Spine 1996;21:945–951.
35. Werneke MW, et al: Clinical effectiveness of behavioral signs for screening chronic low-back pain patients in a work-oriented physical rehabilitation program. Spine 1993;18:2412–2418.
36. Aronoff GM: Editorial Clin J Pain 1985;1(1):1–3.
37. Main CJ, Waddell G: Psychometric construction and validity of the Pilowsky Illness Behavior Questionnaire in British patients with chronic low back pain. Pain 1987;9:13–25.
38. Roland M, Morris R: A study of the natural history of back pain. Part I: Development of a reliable and sensitive measure of disability in low back pain. Spine 1983;8:141–144.
39. Fairbanks J, Couper J, Davies J, O'Brien J: The Oswestry Low Back Pain Disability Questionnaire. Physiotherapy 1980;66:271–273.
40. Roberts A: The conservative treatment of low back pain. MD thesis, University of Nottingham, 1991.
41. Deyo RA: Comparative validity of the sickness impact profile and shorter scales for functional assessment in low back pain. Spine 1986;11:951–954.
42. Gallagher RM: Treating depression in patients with co-morbid pain: Part I. Directions in Psychiatry 1998;18(1):81–97.
43. Gallagher RM: Treating depression in patients with co-morbid pain. Part II. Directions in Psychiatry 1998;18(2):319–335.
44. Romano JH, Turner JA: Chronic pain and depression: Does the evidence support a relationship? Psychol Bull 1985;97:18–34.
45. Atkinson H: Psychopharmacologic agents in the treatment of pain syndromes. In Tollison CD (ed): Handbook of Chronic Pain Management. Baltimore, Williams & Wilkins, 1989, pp 69–99.
46. Lindsay PG, Wycoff M: The depression-pain syndrome and its response to antidepressants. Psychosomatics 1981;22:571–577.
47. Magni G, Moreschi C, Rigatti-Luchini S, Merskey H: Prospective study on the relationship between depressive symptoms and chronic musculoskeletal pain. Pain 1994;56:289–207.
48. Gallagher RM, Williams RA, Skelly J, et al: Workers compensation and return to work in low back pain. Pain 1995;61:299–307.
49. Kulick, Ronald J, Baker, William K: A Guide for Psychological Testing and Evaluation for Chronic Pain. Evaluation and Treatment of Chronic Pain, Aronoff GM, Williams & Wilkins.
50. Reitsman B, Miejler WJ: Pain and patienthood. Clin J Pain 1997;13:9–21.
51. Jensen MP, Karoly P, Huger P: The development and preliminary validation of an instrument to assess patients' attitudes toward pain. J Psychosom Res 1987;31:393–400.
52. Hazard R, et al: Early prediction of chronic disability after occupational low back injury. Spine 1996;21:945–951.
53. Feldman J, (1998) The Workers' Compensation Patient: A Paradoxical Cognitive-Behavioral Approach to Rehabilitation, Current Review of Pain, Aronoff GM, Volume 2, Number 1, 1998.
54. Lancourt J, & Kettelhut M. (1992) Predicting return to work for lower back pain patients receiving workers' compensation. Spine 17:629–640.
55. Tate DG (1992). Workers disability and return to work. American Journal of Physical Medicine and Rehabilitation, 71:92–96.
56. Bigos SJ, et al: A longitudinal, prospective study of industrial back injury reporting. Clin Orthopaed Related Res 1992;279:21–34.
57. Bigos SJ, et al: A prospective study of work perceptions and psychosocial factors affecting the report of back injury. Spine 1991;16:1–6.
58. Feldman J: The Workers' Compensation Patient: A Paradoxical Cognitive-Behavioral Approach to Rehabilitation. Current Review Pain 2(1), 1998.
59. Frank, et al: Disability resulting from occupational low back pain. Part I: What do we know about primary prevention? A review of the scientific evidence on prevention before disability begins. Part II: What do we know about secondary prevention? A review of the scientific evidence on prevention after disability begins. Spine 1996;21:2908–2929.
60. Frank et al: Preventing disability from work-related low-back pain. New evidence gives new hope—if we can just get all the players on side CMAJ, 1998;152(12):1625–1631.
61. Guest GH, Drummond PD. (1992) Effect of compensation on emotional state and disability in chronic back pain. Pain 48:125–130.

62. Cummings N: Psychotherapy and workers' compensation: Golden opportunity or future disgrace? Workshop presented at The Brief Therapy Conference: Essence and Evaluation. Orlando, Florida. December 8–12, 1993. Audiotape available from the Milton H. Erickson Foundation, Phoenix, Az.

63. Mundy RR: Disability syndrome: The effects of early vs. delayed rehabilitation intervention. Am Assoc Occup Health Nursing J, 42:379–383, 1994.

64. Catchclove R, Cohen K: Effects of a directive return to work approach in the treatment of workers' compensation patients with chronic pain. Pain 1982;14:181–191.

65. Hall H, McIntosh G, Melles T, Holowachuk B, & Wai E: Effect of discharge recommendations on outcome. Spine, 1994;(19),2033–2037.

66. Aronoff GM, DuPuy David N: Evaluation and management of back pain: preventing disability. J Back Musculoskel Rehabil 1997;9:109–124.

67. Matheson LN: Work Capacity Evaluation. Trabuco Canyon, CA, ERIC Publishing, 1987.

68. Lechner DE: Functional Capacity Evaluation. In Sourcebook of Occupational Rehabilitation, edited by Phyllis M. King. New York, NY, Plenum Press, 1998.

69. Fishbain D, et al: Physician limitations when assessing work capacity: A review, J Back Musculoskel Rehabil 5:2 (1995):107–113.

70. King PM: A Critical Review of Functional Capacity Evaluations, Physical Therapy Volume 1998;8:852–865.

71. Isernhagen SJ: Functional Capacity Evaluation: rationale, procedure, and utility of the kinesiological approach. Journal of occupational Rehabilitation. 1992;2:157–164.

72. Tramposh AK: The functional capacity evaluation: measuring maximal work abilities. Occup Med 1992;7:113–124.

73. Smith RO: Computer-assisted functional assessment and documentation. J Occup Ther 1993;47:988–992.

74. Lecner DE, Bradbury SF, Bradley LA: Detecting sincerity of effort: A summary of methods and approaches. Phys Ther 1998;78:867–888.

JAMES B. TALMAGE, MD

ASSESSMENT AND MANAGEMENT OF UPPER AND LOWER EXTREMITY IMPAIRMENT AND DISABILITY

From Cookeville Regional
  Medical Center
Cookeville, Tennessee

Reprint requests to:
James B. Talmage, MD
Occupational Health Center
A Division of Cookeville Regional
  Medical Center
1245 E. Spring Street, Suite G
Cookeville, TN 38501

The extremities are frequently involved in both occupational and nonoccupational injuries and illnesses. The physicians involved in treating and/or evaluating the individuals with these problems usually possess current knowledge of the diagnosis and treatment of musculoskeletal problems. A number of textbooks are available, some written at a basic level,[1] and some at a specialist level.[2,3,4,5]

Most individuals recover fully, as the human body has vast healing powers, and medical treatment today is effective for most problems. This article addresses the issues of evaluation and management of impairment and disability when there is *incomplete* recovery. Other authors in this volume discuss in more detail the various medical-systems, and how impairment and disability issues are handled in those systems.

The concepts of impairment and disability are similar, but different. According to the *Guides to the Evaluation of Permanent Impairment, 4th edition* (published by the American Medical Association):

> *Impairment is . . . an alteration of an individual's health status. Impairment . . . is assessed by medical means and is a medical issue. An impairment is a deviation from normal in a body part or organ system and its functioning. The Guides defines "permanent impairment" as one that has become static or stabilized during a period of time sufficient to allow optimal tissue repair, and one that is unlikely to change in spite of future medical or surgical therapy.*

The Guides definition of an impairment closely parallels that of the World Health Organization (WHO) which has defined an impairment is "any loss or abnormality of psychological, physiological, or anatomic structure or function."

The *Guides* defines disability as:

... an alteration of an individual's capacity to meet personal, social, or occupational demands, or statutory or regulatory requirements, because of an impairment. Disability refers to an activity or task the individual cannot accomplish. A disability arises out of the interaction between impairment and external requirements, especially those of a person's occupation. Disability may be thought of as the gap between what a person can *do and what the person* needs *or* wants *to do.*

This article will discuss first the assessment of permanent impairment in extremity injuries and illnesses, and then the management or minimization of disability. The assessment of impairment in extremity problems is similar to the assessment of impairment for other body parts or systems. The treating or examining physician needs to record:

- **History**
  Pre-existing problems from prior injury(s) or disease
  Injury mechanism or disease (symptom) onset
  Chronology of medical tests and treatment (including response to treatment)
  Current symptoms
  Impact of current symptoms on activities of daily living
- **Physical Examination**
  Amputations?
  Deformities? Scars? Skin loss?
  Joint range of motion
  Joint instability
  Neurologic exam (motor, sensory, atrophy, reflexes—deep tendon and pathologic)
  Vascular exam (pulses, edema, temperature, color, Raynaud's phenomenon, tissue loss)
  Other abnormalities (e.g., crepitus, impingement, tendon triggering, subluxation)
- **Test Results**
  Imaging studies (x-ray, CT scan, MRI, bone scan, Doppler ultrasound, arteriogram)
  Electrodiagnostic studies (e.g., EMG/NCV)
  Functional capacity testing
- **Consultations**

With this information, the physician prepares to discuss a number of issues, regardless of whether the problem is with an extremity, or the spine, heart, lungs, or any other system or body part. These issues are: (1) **Diagnosis.** Is the individual at maximal medical improvement ? If yes, what maintenance treatment is recommended? If no, what treatment would likely result in improvement? (2) **Causation.** Is the cause of the current symptoms/impairment known within reasonable medical probability (51% of the evidence). Is apportionment among two or more causes appropriate? (3) **Impairment rating.** What system is to be consulted in the impairment rating process? The AMA *Guides,* or a state-specific worker's compensation system, or FELA? (4) **Abilities** (capacities) and **restrictions** (risk assessment).

ASSESSMENT OF IMPAIRMENT

Diagnosis

When major organizations have published criteria for a diagnosis, those criteria should be followed and referenced (for example, American College of Rheumatology criteria for rheumatoid arthritis). While diagnosis may be straightforward in some cases (fracture of the distal radius and ulna), it can be unclear in others. In worker's compensation for example, many individuals with "repetitive jobs" have subjective symptoms of pain and/or numbness, but either no objective findings, or findings that do not permit a consensus as to the diagnosis. Different physicians may choose to use different terms to describe the same condition, without clear definitions of the terms being used. An example is the study on nonmenclature by Fardon et al.[6] Fifty-one spine surgeons were asked to list the four most common diagnoses they saw in their practices. The authors received 50 different terms:

- Nonspecific/pain syndromes
  Deconditioning syndrome
  Facet syndrome
  Idiopathic lumbar pain
  Low back pain
  Lumbago
  Lumbar pain syndrome
  Mechanical derangement
  Sciatica
- Disc specific disorders
  Degenerative disc disease
  Degenerative disc syndrome
  Disc disease
  Disc disruption
  Disc herniation
  Disc protrusion
  Herniated nucleus pulposis
  Internal disc derangement
  Internal disc disorder
- Degenerative and arthritic
  Arthritis
  Degenerative arthritis
  Degenerative joint disease
  Degenerative spine disease
  Facet arthritis
  Facet arthrosis
  Fascetitis
  Facet spondylosis

Hypertrophic arthritis
Spondylosis
- Muscle/tendon disorder
  Acute and chronic sprain
  Fibromyositis
  Sprain
  Sprain/strain
  Strain
  Tendinitis
- Stability
  Degenerative instability
  Lumbar (spinal) instability
  Segmental instability
- Stenosis
  Central stenosis
  Stenosis
- Miscellaneous
  Failed low back surgery
  Fracture
  Nerve root compression
  Osteoporosis
  Post laminectomy syndrome
  Pseudoarthrosis
  Radiculopathy
  Scoliosis
  Spondylolisthesis
  Spondylolysis

In the extremities, as in the spine, communication is hampered when different practioners use various (undefined) terms to describe the same patient. The increasingly frequent requirement of third party payers for an ICD-9 diagnosis number with each office visit bill may force some degree of common term usage over time, but the ICD-9 book does not state criteria for each diagnosis.

In addition, some physicians use a specific diagnosis label for unexplained symptoms. For example, the term "tendinitis" is frequently diagnosed when pain is present, but without objective evidence of tendon pathology. When the diagnosis is not objectively documented, a better choice is to use a descriptive term for the symptom—for example, "pain in the arm" (ICD-9 code 729.5), "numbness" (782.0), "swelling of limb" (729.81), or "unspecified disorder of muscle, ligament, and fascia" (728.9).

Weiland, who at the time was president of the American Society for Surgery of the Hand, wrote:

> *Tendinitis is a term that clearly indicates inflammation of tendons or tendon-muscle attachments, while tenosynovitis indicates inflammation of a tendon sheath. These terms are examples of clearly definable and diagnosable entities with a known histologic appearance. In the absence of edema, erythema, or crepitation, it is inappropriate to assign the provisional diagnosis of tendinitis or tenosynovitis to patients with upper extremity pain. If patients are told they have one of these conditions, the oppressive power of these words may lead them to believe they are severely injured. A treating physician would do better to explain to their patients that they have pain or fatigue that may or may not be related to their occupation, but there is no definable diagnosis.[7]*

Descriptive terms that imply a possible cause (for example, repetitive strain injury or cumulative trauma disorder) should not be used as a diagnosis. In that same editorial, Weiland states:

> *The American Society for Surgery of the Hand is concerned that patients with upper extremity pain are being assigned specific diagnoses on the basis of subjective complaints without objective physical findings. There is also a tendency to assign a causal relationship to work for this pain when there is a lack of epidermiological evidence. As part of our normal process of providing the best care for our patients, it is important that the diagnosis be accurate and the assignment of causation be correct. The American Society for Surgery of the Hand feels that the diagnoses of "cumulative trauma disorder" (CTD) and "repetitive strain disorder" (RSI) are not appropriate and may actually lead the patient to believe that he or she has a condition that is something more than the ordinary aches and pains of life.*

If objective findings do not permit a consensus as to what is wrong (diagnosis), then scientific agreement on causation is probably impossible. In addition, history may prove ideas of causation to be incorrect. In the first 16 years following the 1884 initiation of the first worker's compensation system in Germany, approximately 2000 books and papers were published on "traumatic cancer."[8] In Great Britain, long after the telegraph came into common usage, "telegrapher's wrist" or "telegraphist's cramp" became a popular diagnosis. After this diagnosis was added to the schedule of compensable illnesses, an epidemic occurred, with 60% of telegraph operators becoming affected. "A committee formed to investigate the condition concluded that those so affected were of a decidedly nervous temperament. The complaints from this activity gradually declined."[8] This epidemic rise and subsequent decline occurred with no change in the working conditions for the telegraph operators.

Another example of time and history correcting popular but erroneous diagnoses is the Australian "repetition strain injury" epidemic of the early 1980s. An Australian hand surgeon reviewed the epidemic in a 1995 article in the *Journal of Hand Surgery*.[9] This epidemic involved complaints of arm pain which both the patient and initial healthcare providers thought were caused by repetitive strain or activity in the workplace. Once the diagnosis became publicized by the media, it became an epidemic involving a large percentage of the working population. "This phenomenon became so prevalent that those of us dealing in upper limb disorders were overwhelmed to the exclusion of the normal practice of hand surgery."[9] The workers had symptoms, but the symptoms didn't fit any known condition, and there were no objective findings. The epidemic ended relatively abruptly when two things happened. First, the Australian physicians, who had previously certified these patients as injured and in need of treatment and rest (which proved to be ineffective), in response to research, began to consider RSI an occupational neurosis." Second, the Supreme Court of Australia ruled in several cases that the employers were not guilty of negligence and the plaintiffs had not suffered injuries. The costs involved were assessed to the plaintiffs.[9]

These historical examples show what can happen when physicians make up a diagnostic name for symptoms, and choose a name that implies known causation. When multiple physicians have seen the same patient, and listed different diagnoses, this suggests that:

1. The patient has had different problems at different points in time.
2. The patient has had the same problem when evaluated by different physicians, but the physicians use different synonymous terms for the same objectively documentable problem ("Colles fracture" and "fracture of the distal radius and ulna").
3. The patient has symptoms, but no objectively documentable problem, leading to multiple speculative "diagnoses."

An accurate and objectively verifiable diagnosis is important for several reasons. At times the diagnosis will determine compensability. For example, in Virginia and in most European countries, carpal tunnel syndrome is not compensable in the worker's compensation system.[10] England and Australia have passed legislation prohibiting claims for compensation and disability unless they are based on objective findings.[11] Similarly, hand and wrist pain attributed to rheumatoid arthritis, Dupuytren's contracture, or to Kienböck's disease are not compensable in worker's compensation systems, since these are diseases with unknown causes.

Treatment recommendations logically depend on an accurate diagnosis. Some medical treatment is symptom directed, i.e., chosen to modify a specific symptom (e.g., aspirin for fever). When a specific diagnosis is known, in general, treatment is more specific and more efficacious. Risk assessment or physician-imposed activity restrictions must be based on an accurate diagnosis.

MAXIMAL MEDICAL IMPROVEMENT

The next issue for the impairment rating physician to prepare to discuss is the concept of maximal medical improvement (MMI). This is the point in time when the individual's problem has stabilized or become permanent. According to the AMA *Guides,* the individual's condition or impairment "is considered to be unlikely to change substantially and by more than 3% in the next year with or without medical treatment."[12] Part of the knowledge base required for this determination is an understanding of the usual healing times for various injuries. Most fractures in the extremities heal in 6–12 weeks. Fractures of the tibia may take 6 months, and at times tibial fractures heal with delayed union, requiring even 12 months to achieve healing. Usually, delayed fracture healing is recognized (x-ray studies permit an objective assessment) and treated with surgery (fixation, bone grafting) and/or some form of electric stimulation. Acute soft tissue injuries to ligaments, muscles, and tendons usually heal in 3–6 weeks for mild to moderate injuries, and in 12 weeks or less for more severe injuries. The fracture concepts of "delayed union" and "non-union" have no correlate in soft tissue conditions. Scar forms consistently. Scar may not properly reconstitute the injured structure, but scar forms consistently in the first weeks following injury.

In chronic tendinitis, consideration of surgical treatment is generally recommended after 4–6 months of conservative treatment. If the tendinitis is going to heal (and it usually does), it should have healed by this point in time.[13]

Thus, most extremity problems will have recovered and be at MMI by 3–6 months after injury, onset, or last surgery. Many states have a legal concept of "statute of limitations" of 1 year following injury. This 1-year interval is based on the assumption that the injured party knows in a year or less if he or she has recovered without sequelae, or with permanent impairment, so the injured party can decide within a year of the injury whether or not to bring a lawsuit for damages.

When the individual with an extremity problem has both stable (unchanging) symptoms and examination findings, and an adequate "healing time" since onset/injury has occurred, the individual is at MMI unless new treatment can be offered and accepted that is likely to change the impairment. A dilemma for physicians is whether or not to offer new, evolving, or perhaps experimental treatment when the patient seems to be at MMI after conventional treatment. Consider, for example, the knee. For the individual with an osteochondral fracture, osteochondritis dissecans, or localized osteoarthritis, all of which leave a full-thickness cartilage defect on the articular surfaces, traditional therapy with nonsteroidal anti-inflammatory drugs and physical therapy is not very helpful. Two new surgical procedures, autogenous cartilage implantation and autogenous osteochondral grafting, have been reported in short-term outcome studies to be beneficial.[14] Deciding when enough research has been done on new procedures so that they can be recommended to patients as evolving standard treatment is quite difficult.[15]

Causation

Causation is a legal concept. Most medical school training is in disease or injury recognition and treatment, with little instruction time spent on the issue of causation. In some disability systems (for example, social security disability), causation is not an issue. In these systems, disability is disability, regardless of the cause of the individual's inability to work. In other legal systems, causation is a critical issue (for example, worker's compensation and personal injury tort litigation). The decision on causation determines whether or not the condition is compensable. If it is ruled noncompensable, then the administrative rules of that system do not apply to impairment and/or disability assessment.

With acute injuries, causation is usually obvious. "In all reasonable medical probability (51% of the evidence), his fall from the third story of the building under construction was the cause of his broken femur." If extremity pain and/or numbness are the symptoms in an individual with a repetitive job, the issue of causation is difficult, if not impossible, to answer with scientific precision. NIOSH has published a text, *A Guide to the Work-Relatedness of Disease, Revised Edition,* January 1979 (PB-298 561), which states:

> *In the current worker's compensation system, the end result of the adjudicatory process is a decision the claimant (employee) has or has not established that he has an occupational disease, that is, a disease condition resulting from, or aggravated by, his employment. The first consideration in determining the probability of a cause/effect relationship between an illness and an agent at the workplace is to establish:*
> 1. *That the disease condition does in fact exist, and*
> 2. *That the particular manifestations of the disease appear to be the result of exposure to a specific harmful agent.*
>   *It would be convenient if a method could be devised which invariably led to a correct and unequivocal decision regarding the presence of an occupation disease. However, it*

is doubtful that such a system could be developed. A case in which the relationship of an illness to a documented agent exposure is clearly evident is not apt to be contested or to require the mechanism of a formal claims inquiry. On the other hand, decision-making may be extremely difficult in many contested claims. Honest differences of opinions are common, "facts" may be subject to different interpretations, and considerable judgment is necessary when data are lacking or incomplete.

Thus, NIOSH seems to be saying that the more disputed the issue of causation, the less scientific the answer is likely to be. In the 21 years since the publication of that document, there is still no scientific method to decide causation. Again, in worker's compensation and personal injury systems, causation is a legal determination, not necessarily a medically proven fact. For example, many states have "heart laws." These laws state that all heart attacks and strokes occurring in policemen and firemen are legally presumed to have been caused by occupational stress (and are therefore covered by worker's compensation), unless the employer can present clear and compelling evidence to the contrary. This makes no scientific sense, yet it has been passed into law by many state legislatures. Similarly, cigarettes are estimated to have killed over 400,000 Americans each and every year, yet no cigarette manufacturer has ever paid a product liability damage award.

The lack of scientific certainty to causation decisions in extremity impairment and disability cases explains why, in the same case (same facts), well-qualified physicians testify that work definitely caused a worker's problem, while other equally qualified physicians testify that there is no scientific way to say that the worker's job caused the problem in question. For physicians who are unfamiliar with the details of medical-legal causation assessment, the first few chapters of *Occupational Medicine Practice Guidelines: Evaluation and Management of Common Health Problems and Functional Recovery in Workers*, published by the American College of Occupational and Environment Medicine offer a concise review.

The issue of the work-relatedness of upper extremity symptoms (cumulative trauma disorders) is crucial. This is discussed well in Kasdan's book *Occupational Hand & Upper Extremity Injuries & Diseases*[2]:

The many disorders that are linked to cumulative trauma can and do occur as regional musculoskeletal illnesses with no provoking activity or cause, making it difficult to determine work-relatedness. Because determination of work-relatedness has far-reaching consequences, the available scientific knowledge, however sparse, is crucial in making a determination. The illness or injury should correlate with the work activities, and symptoms and findings should correlate with the pathophysiology and the time of symptom onset.

While work-relatedness is a legal decision made in most states by the insurance company, determination frequently is influenced by the treating physician's opinion and documentation. To wrongly imply that a musculoskeletal illness is work-related increases the likelihood of disability developing; inappropriately excludes an individual from his job, affecting him both emotionally and financially; and adds and unnecessary financial drain on the workers' compensation system. Such errors may misdirect medical care and lead to unnecessary lost time. On the other hand, to not appropriately recognize a condition as being work-induced can lead to a prolonged course and impairment, as well as deny the patient the workers' compensation to which he or she is entitled.

The problem is compounded by an older workforce that is experiencing the chronic, degenerative musculoskeletal effects of aging and by the overall increasingly deconditioned state of all age groups of workers. The aches and pains of aging, deconditioning, and poor posture might all too easily be attributed to work-related activities. Another factor to consider is that presently in the United States, psychiatric disorders are not reimbursed by insurance companies at as high a percentage as physical diseases, making it economically advantageous for both patient and physician to interpret symptoms as reflecting physical disease rather than emotional distress or mental illness. The current structure of the "no fault" workers' compensation system allows many opportunities for primary and secondary gain issues to complicate diagnosis and treatment and to delay recovery.

Carpal tunnel syndrome (CTS) is a common musculoskeletal illness that illustrates the difficulties involved in causation issues. CTS is the symptom complex of numbness (with or without pain) in the distribution of the median nerve in the hand. Entrapment of the median nerve at the wrist (in the carpal tunnel) is the suspected pathology. Causation decisions are extremely complex, as this condition has been statistically associated with a number of diseases[16,17,18,19,20] and with some occupations.[21,22,23] In addition, many cases are idiopathic.[16]

Medical conditions that have been statistically associated with CTS include: (1) those that narrow the carpal tunnel, including wrist fracture, tumor, infections, aberrant muscles, flexor tenosynovitis (nonspecific as well as that associated with rheumatoid arthritis[16]), and congenitally small carpal tunnels.[24] (2) systemic conditions such as pregnancy, obesity, diabetes mellitus, hypothyroidism, inflammatory arthritis, alcoholism, smoking, hemodialysis, a sedentary lifestyle, and amyloidosis.[5,16]

A number of work-related factors have been statistically associated with CTS. Many of the studies involved can be criticized for defining an individual as having CTS based on symptoms and subjective physical exam findings (without benefit of the only known objective test for this problem, nerve conduction testing or electrodiagnostic testing). The usually stated risk factors for occupational repetitive motion disorders are[25]:

- High repetitions: jobs with a cycle time of less than 30 seconds, or more than 50% of the cycle time involved in performing fundamentally the same cycle or activity.
- High force: jobs in which the *estimated* average hand force requirements are more than 4 kg. (There still is no good way to measure actual hand grip forces used on most jobs.)
- Awkward wrist posture: posturing in more than 45 degrees of wrist flexion or extension, without excessive radial or ulnar deviation.
- Use of vibrating power tools (not clearly defined).

Attempting to define the role of work in the causation of CTS has been the topic of many articles, and even book chapters.[10,20,22] One of the best reviews of this subject is found in Kasdan's book.[23] This review of the best data suggests that " . . . neither force nor repetition alone increases the risk for median nerve slowing, but in combination the odds ratio is 1.95 (95% confidence interval 1.3–3.4)." This means that jobs with high force and repetition essentially double the risk of CTS.

While epidemiological data may permit statements like: "Smoking doubles the risk of heart attack," "Diabetes doubles the risk of carpal tunnel syndrome," and "Highly repetitious, highly forceful use of the hands doubles the risk for carpal tunnel syndrome," they apply to populations and not to individuals. If an individual who smokes has a heart attack, there is a 50% chance that the heart attack would have occurred even if he or she were a nonsmoker. If a woman with diabetes develops CTS, there is a 50% chance she would have developed it even if she were not diabetic. Similarly, if CTS develops in a worker with a job requiring highly repetitious and highly forceful work with the hands, there is a 50% chance CTS would have developed even if he had never done that job. In a single individual, no known test can sort out which disease was actually caused by the condition with which it is statistically associated. Yet this is the question that is asked of the treating or evaluating physician in these cases.

Szabo, who had authored chapters on the work-relatedness of carpal tunnel syndrome in several texts,[10] has concluded: "Even if a patient experiences symptoms only at work, an honest clinician is still unable to describe the extent to which the patient's CTS is related to the job." He continues: "It is unfortunate that worker's compensation determinations must be made in individual cases, where it is impossible to quantify the contribution of the job to the clinical problem." Nevertheless, OSHA has concluded that there is enough epidemiological evidence for work-relatedness of many musculoskeletal conditions to justify publication of a working draft of OSHA's proposed ergonomics standard.[26]

Given the same facts, different administrative systems have reached different conclusions. In the United States, CTS is considered potentially caused by work, and therefore potentially compensable under worker's compensation. The exception is Virginia, where House Bill 2556, effective 7/1/97, states: " . . . and the condition of carpal tunnel syndrome are not occupational diseases but are ordinary diseases of life as defined in section 65.2-401." Similarly, in most of the rest of the world, CTS is not considered a work-related disorder.[10] In addition to the decision on causation of CTS determining whether or not the rules of an administrative system (like worker's compensation) apply to an individual case, the decision on causation may affect the prognosis. Similar to the studies on low back pain, studies have shown that the prognosis (or treatment result) in CTS is worse if the condition is considered work-related, than if the condition is considered not work-related.[27,28]

Finally, before leaving the question of causation in carpal tunnel syndrome, note the obvious paradox in the question. A syndrome is defined as: "a set of symptoms which occur together; the sum of signs of any morbid state; a symptom complex."[29] In the history of medicine, conditions that have an unknown basis frequently are first referred to as syndromes, to denote the pattern of symptoms seen. When, with research over time, the pathophysiology of the condition (and thus cause) becomes known, the condition is usually renamed. Thus, what was at first referred to as "Down's syndrome" later became known as "trisomy 21." Thus, to state the cause of CTS as a known fact, is to state the cause of a group of symptoms that occur together but which, by definition, have no known cause.

Because carpal tunnel syndrome is common, and causation is controversial, there is a fair amount of research on this topic. The other illnesses of the upper and lower extremities that are suspected of being work-related are much less well researched. This makes determination of causation in these cases even more problematic. There is some evidence of statistical association between work activities and a number of musculoskeletal disorders. This list would include at least rotator cuff tendinitis, de Quervain's tenosynovitis, and trigger finger/thumb.

Some conditions are commonly misperceived as work-related. For example, lateral epicondylitis of the elbow is discussed as if it were work-related in some texts. A review of the available literature caused the authors of the American College of Occupational and Environmental Medicine *Occupational Medicine Practice Guidelines* to conclude that the "strength of association/odds ratio" was "not significant."[30] The next *Musculoskeletal Disorders in the Workplace: Principles and Practice* devotes individual chapters to low back, neck, shoulder, wrist and hand, knee and hip, foot and ankle, etc. disorders. This text does not have a chapter on the elbow, but simply states: "Work-related musculoskeletal ailments of the elbow are rare. The conditions of a painful elbow joint can be worsened by repetitive work, but the primary origins of the disorder should first be attended. The clinical syndrome of this joint will not be discussed in this text."[31] A good discussion of erroneous links to work is found in Kasdan's book[32]:

A number of medical conditions of the upper extremity often are mistakenly assumed to be caused by work. Frequently the patient has great difficulty understanding and accepting that the problem would have developed regardless of the type of work performed. Os-

teoarthritis of the hands, particularly basal thumb joint and finger joint arthritis, may be inappropriately labeled as work-related. Neither Heberden's nodules or Dupuytren's contractures are found to correlate with work stress. Ulna carpal abutment, caused by a congenital, excessively long ulna abutting against the carpal bones, may cause significant symptoms of wrist pain with use, and can be inappropriately ascribed to work activities.

Ganglions of the hand and wrist are common, but the cause is unknown. Theories include underlying carpal bone instability and degenerative processes. Despite lack of epidemiological evidence of work-relatedness, ganglions are frequently considered by insurance carriers as being caused by work if the patient complains of symptoms with work-related activities. Fibromyalgia pain syndrome, which is defined by a lack of objective findings and the presence of pain, occasionally is presented as being work-related despite any supporting data in the literature.

Thus, physicians are frequently asked to determine the causation of extremity disorders, in spite of lack of scientific methods for such determinations. The causation decision affects compensability, the appropriateness of work restrictions, and the prognosis for treatment, so it is a crucially important decision.

Impairment Rating

Rating permanent impairment is one of the issues the treating or evaluating physician must be prepared to deal with in extremity injury and disease cases. In worker's compensation cases this is usually a requirement of the state law. In personal injury and disability assessment cases, the impairment rating is much less important and may not even have a role. Rating permanent impairment is an attempt to describe the consequences of an injury or disease(s) by using a number. Instead of saying "mild" or "severe," the physician uses a system to numerically rate anatomic, physiologic, and psychologic consequences of the problem. One of the various editions of the *Guides to the Evaluation of Permanent Impairment* is used in many states worker's compensation systems. Some states have written their own systems for rating impairment in worker's compensation. In all of these states, the impairment rating helps the system determine what level of compensation and benefits to award to the injured worker.

The medical basis for the impairment rating in extremity cases is a complete history and physical exam, supplemented at times by appropriate imaging or lab studies. The impairment rating physician needs to know the administrative system in which a particular case is pending so that appropriate and complete medical data necessary for the assessment are acquired. For example, if the 4th edition of the *AMA Guides* is to be used, there is a checklist for completeness of the examination (see Tables 1 and 2).

As medical science advances, permanent impairment rating systems change—although usually years after new treatment protocols and new scenarios in need of rating are seen. Newer surgical procedures such as autogenous cartilage implantation and autogenous osteochondral grafting, as well as surgical replacement of torn cruciate ligaments and menisci with allografts[36] represent examples of scenarios that may require impairment rating, but that are not mentioned in the impairment rating system.

The process of rating permanent impairment is fairly complex, and is specific to the administrative system in question. If additional information on the process of impairment rating (and disability assessment) is desired, the following organizations conduct continuing medical education courses for physicians on this topic:

American Academy of Disability Evaluating Physicians, tel. 800-456-6095

American Academy of Physical Medicine and Rehabilitation, tel. 312-464-9700

American College of Occupational and Environmental Medicine, tel. 847-228-6850 ext. 184

National Association of Disability Evaluating Professionals, tel. 804-378-8809

SEAK, Inc.-Medical and Legal Information Systems, tel. 508-457-1111

TABLE 1.   Checklist for Upper Extremity Impairment Evaluations*

Amputation Present?	Rate By	
Thumb	Figure 7 (26)	
Finger(s)	Figure 17 (30)	
More proximal	Figure 2 (18)	

Range of Motion Measured?	Rate By	As Shown In
Thumb IP, flexion/extension	Figure 10 (26)	Figure 8 (25)
MP, flexion/extension	Figure 13 (27)	Figure 11 (27)
CMC adduction (cm)	Table 5 (28)	Figure 14 (28)
radial abduction	Table 6 (28)	Figure 15 (29)
opposition (cm)	Table 7 (29)	Figure 16 (29)
Finger(s) DIP, flexion/extension	Figure 19 (32)	Figure 18 (32)
PIP, flexion/extension	Figure 21 (33)	Figure 20 (33)
MP, flexion/extension	Figure 23 (34)	Figure 22 (34)
Wrist, flexion/extension	Figure 26 (36)	Figure 24 (36)
radial/ulnar deviation	Figure 29 (28)	Figure 27 (37)
Elbow, flexion/extension	Figure 32 (40)	Figure 30 (39)
pronation/supination	Figure 35 (41)	Figure 33 (40)
Shoulder, flexion/extension	Figure 38 (43)	Figure 36 (42)
abduction/adduction	Figure 41 (44)	Figure 39 (43)
external/internal rotation	Figure 44 (45)	Figure 42 (44)

Loss of Sensation Present?

Part	Measure	Type of Loss	Level of Injury
Thumb	2 point	Longitudinal (1 nerv˜e)	Figure 7 (24), Table 4 (25)
		Transverse (both nerves)	Figure 7 (24), Figure 7 (24)
Finger (index, middle, or ring)	2 point	Longitudinal (1 nerve)	Figure 17 (30), Table 9 (31)
		Transverse (both nerves)	Figure 17 (30), Figure 17 (30)
Finger (little)	2 point	Longitudinal (1 nerve)	Figure 17 (30), Table 8 (31)
		Transverse (both nerves)	Figure 17 (30), Figure 17 (30)
Hand/wrist—light touch and/or sharp-dull discrimination			
• Median nerve		Palmar cutaneous branch	Figure 45 (50), (22)
• Ulnar nerve		Palmar/dorsal cutaneous branch	Figure 45 (50), (22)
• Radial nerve		Superficial branch(es)	Figure 45 (50), (22)
Upper extremity—light touch and/or sharp-dull discrimination			
• Peripheral nerve		Figure 45 (50), Tables 15 (54) & 11 (48)	
• Spinal nerve		Neurology text, Tables 13 (51) & 11 (48)	
• Brachial plexus		Neurology text, Tables 14 (52) & 11 (48)	

Note: partial impairment to 7- to 15-mm 2-point discrimination, total ≥ 16 mm

Additional Neurologic Signs
  Reflexes: biceps, triceps, brachioradialis
          Pathologic
  Coordination: rapid alternating movements (e.g., button a button, turn pages in a book)

Motor (Muscle) Weakness

Type of Loss	Level of Injury	Impairment
Peripheral nerve	Figure 48 (53)	Table 15 (54) & 12 (49)
Spinal nerve	Neurology text	Tables 13 (51) & 12 (49)
Brachial plexus	Neurology text	Tables 14 (52) & 12 (49)

Table continues on next page.

TABLE 1.   Checklist for Upper Extremity Impairment Evaluations* *(Cont.)*

Peripheral Vascular Injury	
Table 17(57)	**Complex Regional Pain Syndrome**
Pulses	Edema
Edema	Skin color red or purple
Amputation or tissue (pulp) loss	Local dyshidrosis
Temperature (measure)	Abnormal temperature (measure)
Raynaud's phenomenon	Decreased passive motion in joints
	Skin texture: smooth or shiny

Fractures

Measure	Impairment
Crepitus (post-traumatic arthritis)	Table 19 (59) & Table 18 (58)
Digit radial/ulnar deviation	Table 21 (59) & Table 18 (58)
Digit rotational deformity	Table 22 (59) & Table 18 (58)
Wrist/elbow radial/ulnar deformity	Table 25 (60) & Table 18 (58)

Sprains and Dislocations

Measure	Impairment
Presisting subluxation/dislocation	Table 23 (60) & Table 18 (58)
Joint medial/lateral instability	Table 24 (60) & Table 18 (58)
Carpal instability	Table 26 (61)
Extensor tendon subluxation	Table 30 (63) & Table 18 (58)

Inflammatory Disease

Measure	Impairment
Synovial hypertrophy	Table 20 (59) & Table 18 (58)
Wrist radial/ulnar deviation deformity	Table 25 (60) & Table 18 (58)
Intrinsic tightness	Table 28 (63) & Table 18 (58)
Extensor tendon subluxation	Table 30 (63) & Table 18 (58)

Overuse Syndromes

Measure	Impairment
Constrictive tenosynovitis (triggering)	Table 29 (63) & Table 18 (58)
Carpal tunnel syndrome	
Sensation (2-point discrimination)	Tables 15 (54) & 11 (48)
Thumb opposition strength	Tables 15 (54) & 12 (49)

*Page numbers in the *Guides* (4th edition) are indicated in the parentheses.

DISABILITY MANAGEMENT

Abilities and Restrictions

The last area that the treating or evaluating physician needs to consider and discuss in reports (and in treatment, if the physician is in a treating role) is disability, or "abilities and restrictions." Disability is defined by the *AMA Guides, 4th edition* as follows:

> *Disability may be defined as an alteration of an individual's capacity to meet personal, social, or occupational demands, or statutory or regulatory requirements, because of an impairment. Disability refers to an activity or task the individual cannot accomplish. A disability arises out of the interaction between impairment and external requirements, especially those of a person's occupation. Disability may be thought of as the gap between what a person **can** do and what the person **needs** or **wants** to do.*

TABLE 2. Checklist for Lower Extremity Impairment Evaluations*

Condition	Rate By
• *Gate Derangement*	Table 36 (76)
Presence of limp, Trendelenberg sign, arthritis in hip, knee, or ankle	
Use of brace(s), cane(s), crutches, walker, or wheelchair	
• *Limb Length Discrepancy*	Table 35 (75)
By teleroentgenography	
• *Atrophy*	Table 37 (77)
Thigh, measure 10 cm above patella	
Calf, measure maximal circumference	
• *Muscle Weakness*	Table 38–39 (77)
Hip: flexion, extension, abduction	
Knee: flexion, extension	
Ankle: flexion (plantar flexion), extension (dorsiflexion)	
Hind foot: inversion, eversion	
Great toe: extension, flexion	
• *Range of Motion*	
Hip: flexion, extension, internal rotation, external rotation, abduction,	
adduction, abduction contracture,	Table 40 (78)
Knee: flexion, flexion contracture, varus deformity, valgus deformity,	Table 41 (78)
Ankle: plantar flexion, extension/flexion contracture	Table 42 (78)
Hind foot: inversion, eversion	Table 43 (78)
Ankle/hind foot deformity: varus, valgus	Table 44 (78)
Great toe: MTP extension, IP flexion	Table 45 (78)
Lesser toes: MTP extension	
• *Joint Ankylosis*	
Hip	Tables 46–50 (79)
Knee	Table 51–54 (79)
Ankle	Tables 55–59 (80–81)
Toes	Table 61 (82)
Loss of tibia-os-calcis angle	Table 60 (81)
• *Arthritis*	Table 62 (83)
Roentgenographically determined cartilage intervals	
• *Amputations*	Table 63 (83)
Note level of amputation	
• *Diagnosis-Based Estimates*	Table 64 (85–86)
Pelvis, fractures	
Hip, replacement	Table 65 (87)
Femoral neck fracture, girdlestone arthroplasty,	
chronic trochanteric bursitis femoral shaft fracture	Table 65 (87)
Knee: patellar subluxation/instability, fracture	
Patellectomy	
Menisectomy	
Cruciate or collateral ligament laxity	
Plateau fracture	
Supracondylar/intracondylar fracture	
Knee replacement, see also Table 66 (88)	
Proximal tibial osteotomy	
Tibial shaft fracture	
Ankle: ligamentous laxity, fracture	
Hind foot: fracture	
Mid foot/fore foot: deformity	
• *Skin Loss*	Table 67 (88)
Ischium, tibial tuberosity, heel, or plantar surface	
Includes chronic draining osteomyelitis	
• *Nerve Deficits*	
Maximal potential deficit(s); motor, sensory, dysesthesia	Table 68 (89)
Severity multipliers; motor, sensory	Tables 21–20 (151)
• *Peripheral Vascular Disease*	Table 69 (89)
Claudication or rest pain	
Edema, controlled or not by elastic supports	
Pulses	
Loss of subcutaneous tissue	
Arterial calcification by x-ray	
Amputation(s)	

*Page numbers in the *Guides* (4th edition) are indicated in the parentheses.

This definition focuses on the ability of the person to work. Social security disability and, usually, employer-funded or personally funded long-term disability policies focus on whether or not the individual can do any job for which he or she is qualified by training or experience. Social security disability is defined as " . . . the inability to engage in any gainful activity by reason of any medically determinable physical or mental impairment(s) which can be expected to result in death or which has lasted or can be expected to last for a continuous period or not less than 12 months."[37] This definition of total disability also focuses on work ability. An individual may be independent for all activities of daily living done in the home, but still be unable to work.

The two key concepts to remember when discussing work and disability issues are abilities and restrictions. **Abilities** refer to the individual's **capacities to do specific activities.** Capacities can be measured or estimated to some degree. Examples would include measuring the exercise capacity by treadmill testing following a myocardial infarction, or measuring the amount of weight in a crate a person can lift after repair of nerve and tendon lacerations in an upper extremity. Various functional capacity tests are attempts to measure capacity or ability. The reliability, validity, projection to 8-hour workdays, safety protocols, and behavioral assessment of ten commonly used Functional Capacity Assessment systems have recently been reviewed[38]. Unfortunately, all of these issues are problematic for all of these commercially available systems. The difficulty of detecting sincerity of effort in testing (or impairment evaluation situations) has also recently been reviewed[39].

Restrictions refers to physician-suggested activity limitations based on the concept of the **risk the activity in question poses.** Restrictions and risk assessment are not in any way measurable in the individual. In musculoskeletal disorders, physicians recommend restrictions based on some combination of training ("In residency, my chief said always give a 50-pound restriction"), experience ("The last few times I sent someone back to work with a 50-pound restriction . . ."), knowledge of biomechanics, and published medical studies. For low back problems, there is some published literatures on the risk posed by normal activities. For disorders of the extremities, there is little good data on risk assessment, explaining why physician suggestions on permanent restrictions show marked variability.

If a physician's judgement is challenged, according to the Americans with Disabilities Act, to justify permanent restrictions the physician is supposed to have objective evidence that the activity in questions poses a significant risk of substantial harm that is imminent, and cannot be removed or decreased by employer accommodation(s). If a previously painful condition becomes more painful with activity, that does not constitute "significant harm," and the individual may do the activity if he or she wishes.

Most published literature on extremity problem risk assessment (restrictions) is consensus, and not research on what happens in the real world if an individual tries to do certain activities. There is general consensus that some degree of permanent lifting and/or carrying restriction is appropriate for at least the following:

Condition	Risk
Full thickness rotator cuff repairs, whether repaired or unrepairable	Further tear
Avascular necrosis: humeral head, lunate, hip, knee, or ankle (when in lower extremity, subject shouldn't jump down.)	Bone collapse (fracture)
Venous insufficiency	Worse venous insufficiency
Non-united fractures	Increased deformity
Tumors or osteomyelitis of long bones	Fracture

| Paget's disease of bone | Fracture |
| Ligamentous instability of the knee, elbow, wrist, or shoulder | Worse instability |

Another facet of disability evaluation and management involves the issue of when a person may return to work with, or without, temporary restrictions. Again, there is little science to guide the physician when extremity problems are the concern. There is useful information in the following published texts:

- *The Medical Disability Advisor, third edition,* Edited by Presley Reed MD, Published by the Reed Group, Ltd., Boulder, CO (ISBN 0-934753-52-0)
- *Official Disability Guidelines, fourth edition* (1999), published by Work-Loss Data Institute, LLC, Corpus Christi, TX (ISBN 1-880-891-25-5)
- *Occupational Medicine Practice Guidelines: Evaluation and Management of Common Health Problems and Functional Recovery in Workers,* edited by Jeffrey S. Harris MD, published by OEM Press, Beverly, MA (ISBN 1-883595-14-2)

Reed's book lists the duration of disability (time out of work) for approximately 5000 diagnoses or procedures. These tables permit an assessment of when an individual with this problem should be able to return to work, assuming that the job description for the job adequately characterizes the job by *Dictionary of Occupational Titles* criteria. The text also contains line graphs to show the actual duration experience for more than 100 of the most common injuries and illnesses. The real world data come from the combined data bases of *The Medical Disability Advisor* customers, Reed Group disability management service business, and CORE Analytic.

The *Official Disability Guidelines* combines three U.S. government data bases: the Occupational Safety and Health Administration, the Centers for Disease Control, and the National Center for Health Statistics. While providing different data on return-to-work time, this book doesn't consider the difficulty of the job involved, but does provide data for almost all ICD—9 codes.

Harris' book provides consensus recommendations for disability duration for some of the more common conditions that are causes of work absence in worker's compensation and in short-term disability systems. The tables list "Target for Disability Duration with Modified Duty" (with suggested activity modifications and accomodations), as well as "Target for Disability Duration without Modified Duty."

These texts can be consulted and even shown to the person with delayed recovery. Sometimes the knowledge that most folks with similar problems have already returned to work when this far into recovery from injury and/or surgery motivates the individual to return to work.

A comparison shows that the recommendations in Harris' book are a little overly optimistic. Consider, for example, how this text treats ankle sprains:

- Harris' text—Disability duration without modified duty   0–2 days
  - with modified duty   7–21 days
- Reed's text—Sedentary work   Minimum duration   1 day
  - Maximum duration   14 days
  - Heavy/very heavy work   Minimum duration,
    - 1st or 2nd degree   14 days
    - 3rd degree   28 days
    - Maximum duration,
    - 1st or 2nd degree   42 days
    - 3rd degree   112 days
- Data base—Mean observed duration   34 days
  - Median observed duration   23 days

Minimizing Disability

To minimize the disability duration for any illness or injury the treating physician needs to deliver the best, current medical care for the condition. That type of care will be assumed in the remainder of this discussion.

There are injuries and/or diseases in which major impairment of extremity use is permanent. In lower extremity scenarios, ambulation aids and gait training by a therapist are appropriate. When an upper extremity is permanently useless, the individual has to learn to function with only the remaining hand and arm. Mayer's book, *One-Handed in a Two-Handed World,*[40] is an excellent source of information on how to live one-handed. Physicians can recommend the book, or have a copy or two to loan to patients.

Return to work is definitely hastened if the employer will provide modified duty while the injured or ill employee is healing. If the employee feels that he or she cannot return to duty (with or without modification) as defined by the employer, many physicians have found a work site visit—most commonly by a therapist—to be beneficial. The ergonomics of the job can be evaluated to see if additional modification of duties is possible as a compromise the employer and employee can both accept.[38,41] "In workers' compensation, as has been amply shown, prolonged disability is rarely due to the musculoskeletal injury, but is related more to the psychosocial issues that impede a speedy return to work."[42] The work site visit also permits an evaluation of the interpersonal relationship between the patient and other workers, especially supervisors. The best possible "work conditioning" program is probably being at work in modified duty with restrictions that gradually decrease over time. Thus, every effort should be made to negotiate a compromise in work status.

Formal "work conditioning" (4 or more hours a day, 3–5 days a week) featuring specific exercises directed by a therapist may be helpful when work conditioning by working at modified duties is not available. Some jobs (for example, police officer, fire fighter, brick mason) just are not suitable for modified duty.

The last issue to discuss is the hardest—how to motivate the individual with delayed recovery on a psychosocial basis to return to work. As the *AMA Guides* points out, "Motivation is a link between impairment and disability."[43] Delayed recovery in musculoskeletal injury is most frequently due to psychosocial and compensation issues. Thus, extremity problems are similar to low back problems, and require that the treating or evaluating physician be a "generalist" who is able to assess the whole person in addition to the musculoskeletal system. This need is reflected in modern texts. *Occupational Medicine Practice Guidelines*[5] contains Chapter 7: Pain Behavior, Inconsistent Findings, and Motivation for Self-Care and Recovery. *Occupational Hand & Upper Extremity Injuries & Diseases*[2] contains Chapter 2: The Role of Motivation in the Recovery of the Hand, and Chapter 3: Chronic Pain and Suffering: A Sociobiological Problem. *Musculoskeletal Disorders in the Workplace*[3] contains Chapter 6: Psychosocial Aspects of Occupational Musculoskeletal Disorders. *Repetitive Motion Disorders of the Upper Extremity*[4] contains Chapter 37: Overview of Complete Patient Management in Upper Extremity Repetitive Motion Disorders.

Physicians who treat both injured athletes and injured workers are very aware that not all worker's compensation patients have the same motivation to recover that athletes have. What methods are available to the physician to help those patients with extremity injuries or diseases who appear to have significant psychosocial factors that impair recovery? Probably the most important is clear communication. The physician needs to effectively communicate the nature of the physical problem, the limits it imposes on performance, and a realistic prognosis for future ability and symptoms. If the patient has major psychosocial issues impairing recovery, he or she is frequently in denial (ego defense mechanism), and therefore the physician may not be believed. Communication may break through the denial if it is repeated and if information is conveyed in a manner that shows respect and interest in the patient's recovery. Part of repeating the communication is to see that others involved communicate the same, consistent message. Communication between the treating physician and the therapist, between the physician and the case manager, and between the physician and the employer is necessary so that all involved in the case have the same message for the patient.

Appeals to the pride of the individual ("I have quadriplegic patients who work every day") generally are not motivational. Praise, approval, and constant encouragement are more often helpful. If the pain behavior, or apparent lack of motivation for recovery persist, exploration and treatment of psychosocial factors may be the only logical option. Unfortunately, many worker's compensation systems do not want the treating or evaluating physician to consider anything other than the musculoskeletal injury or disease. Referral to the company's employee assistance program, or, if the individual is religious, referral to his or her minister, priest, rabbi, etc. may be helpful. Many of these patients are in denial and can't consciously acknowledge that there are major psychosocial stressors in their lives. Without some degree of emotional insight, psychologic counseling will not be effective. Antidepressant medications may improve the patient's mood and pain, but rarely do they make a difference in motivation to return to work.

The remaining option is to place the individual in a multi-disciplinary treatment program, also known as "tertiary rehabilitation." This type of program uses physical reconditioning and behavioral methods, involving physicians of multiple specialties, as well as psychologists, occupational and physical therapists, and vocational rehabilitation experts. While this type of program is more commonly used in low back pain, success from this method has been reported for upper extremity disorder patients.[44]

Finally, some patients will remain disabled, either by severe physical problems or by minor physical problems coupled with major psychosocial issues. If the individual has no conscious or subconscious motivation to recover and function, treatment may prove to be futile.

CONCLUSION

Impairment and disability issues in extremity disorders are basically the same issue faced by physicians and patients with problems in other body systems. Diagnosis, maximal medical improvement (treatment), causation, impairment rating, and ability assessment/restriction are the issues that concern physicians, insurers, and patients.

REFERENCES

1. Snider RK: Essentials of Musculoskeletal Care. American Academy of Orthopedic Surgeons, Rosemont, Illinois, 1997.
2. Kasdan ML: Occupational Hand & Upper Extremity Injuries & Diseases, 2nd ed. Hanley & Belfus, Inc., Philadelphia, PA, 1998.
3. Nordin M, Andersson GBJ, Pope MH: Musculoskeletal Disorders in the Workplace: Principles and Practice. Mosby, St. Louis, MO, 1997.
4. Gordon SL, Blair SJ, Fine LJ: Repetitive Motion Disorders of the Upper Extremity. American Academy of Orthopedic Surgeons, Rosemont IL, 1995.
5. Harris JS: Occupational Medicine Practice Guidelines. OEM Press, Beverly, MA, 1997.
6. Fardon D, Pinkerton S, Balderston R, et al: Terms used for diagnosis by English-speaking spine surgeons. Spine 18:274–277, 1993.
7. Weiland AJ: Editorial: Repetitive strain injuries and cumulative trauma disorders. J Hand Surg 21:337, 1996.
8. Louis DS: The Still-Evolving History of Compensation for Bodily Harm. In Kasdan ML (ed): Occupational Hand & Upper Extremity Injuries & Diseases, 2nd ed., Hanley & Belfus, Philadelphia, PA, 1998.

9. Ireland DCR: Repetition strain injury: The Australian experience—1992 update. J Hand Surg 20A:S53–S56, 1995

10. Szabo RM, Madison M: Carpal tunnel syndrome as a work-related disorder. In Repetitive Motion Disorders of the Upper Extremity, American Academy of Orthopedic Surgeons, Rosemont, IL, 1995, pp 421–434.

11. Lister G: Ergonomic disorders—An editorial. J Hand Surg (Am) 20 (3):353, 1995.

12. Guides to the Evaluation of Permanent Impairment, 4th ed. The American Medical Association, Chicago, IL, 1993, 315.

13. Almekinders L: Tendinitis and other chronic tendinopathies. J Am Acad Orthop Surg 6:157–164, 1998

14. LaPrade RF, Swiontkowski MF: New horizons in the treatment of osteoarthritis of the knee. J Am Med Ass 281:876–878, 1999.

15. Eddy DM: Clinical decision making: From theory to practice, investigational treatments, how strict should we be? J Am Med Assoc 278:179–185, 1997.

16. Carpal Tunnel Syndrome. The American Academy of Orthopaedic Surgeons Bulletin:4–6, October 1989

17. Kasdan ML, Wolens D, Leis VM, Kasdan AS, Stallings P: Carpal tunnel syndrome not always work related. Kentucky Med J 92:295–297, 1994.

18. Miller RS, Iverson DC, Fried RA, Green LA, Nutting PA: Carpal tunnel syndrome in primary care: A report from ambulatory sentinel practice network. J Fam Prac 38:337–344, 1994.

19. Atcheson SG, Ward JR, Wing Lowe: Concurrent medical disease in work-related carpal tunnel syndrome. Arch Int Med 158:1506–1512, 1998.

20. Nathen PA, Keniston RC: Carpal tunnel syndrome: Personal risk profile and role of intrinsic and behavioral factors. In Kasdan ML (ed): Occupational Hand & Upper Extremity Injuries & Diseases. Hanley & Belfus, Philadelphia, PA, 1998, pp 129–140.

21. Reference deleted.

22. Cannon LJ, Bernacki EJ, Walter SD: Personal and occupational factors associated with carpal tunnel syndrome. J Occup Med 23:255–258, 1981.

23. Szabo RM: Occupational carpal tunnel syndrome. In Kasdan ML (ed): Occupational Hand & Upper Extremity Injuries & Diseases. 2nd ed. Hanley & Belfus, Philadelphia, PA, 1998, pp 113–128.

24. Bleecker ML, Bohlman M, Moreland R, Tipton A: Carpal tunnel syndrome: Role of carpal canal size. Neurology 35:1599–1604, 1985.

25. Silverstein BA, Fine LJ, Armstrong TJ: Occupational factors and carpal tunnel syndrome. Am J Ind Med 11:343–358, 1987.

26. Working Draft of a Proposed Ergonomics Program Standard. http://www.osha-slc.gov/SLTC/ergonomics/ergoreg.html

27. Higgs PE, Edwards D, Martin DS, Weeks PM: Carpal tunnel surgery outcomes in workers: Effect of worker's compensation status. J Hand Surg 20A:354–360, 1995.

28. Al-Qattan MM, Bowen V, Manktelow RT: Factors associated with poor outcome following primary carpal tunnel release in non-diabetic patients. J Hand Surg 19B:622–625, 1994.

29. Dorland's Illustrated Medical Dictionary, 27th ed. W.B. Saunders Company, Philadelphia PA, 1988.

30. Harris JS: Occupational Medicine Practice Guidelines. OEM Press, Beverly, MA, 1997.

31. Nordin M, Andersson GBJ, Pope MH: Musculoskeletal Disorders in the Workplace: Principles and Practice. Mosby, St. Louis, MO, 1997. Page 329.

32. Kasdan ML: Occupational Hand & Upper Extremity Injuries & Diseases, 2nd ed. Hanley & Belfus, Inc., Philadelphia, PA, 1998, p 56.

33. Reference deleted.

34. Reference deleted.

35. Reference deleted.

36. Shelton WR, Treacy SH, Dukes AD, Bomboy AL: Use of allografts in knee reconstruction. J Am Acad Orthop Surg 6:165–175, 1998.

37. Disability Evaluation Under Social Security. SSA Publication No. 64-039, September 1994.

38. King PM, Tuckwell N, Barrett TE: A critical review of functional capacity evaluations. Physical Therapy 78:852–866, 1998.

39. Lechner DE, Bradbury SF, Bradley LA: Detecting sincerity of effort: A summary of methods and approaches. Physical Therapy 78:867–888, 1998.

40. Mayer T-K: One-Handed in a Two-Handed World. Prince-Gallison Press, Boston, MA, 1996.

41. Kasdan ML: Occupational Hand & Upper Extremity Injuries & Diseases, 2nd ed. Hanley & Belfus, Inc., Philadelphia, PA, 1998, p 104.

42. Millender LH, Conlon M: An approach to work-related disorders of the upper extremity. J Am Acad Orthop Surg 4:134–142, 1996.

43. Guides to the Evaluation of Permanent Impairment, 4th ed. American Medical Association, Chicago, IL, 1993, p 298.

44. Feuerstein M: A multidisciplinary approach to the prevention, evaluation, and management of work disability. J Occup Rehabil 1:5–12, 1991.

DONALD E. SHREY, PhD, CRC

WORKSITE DISABILITY MANAGEMENT MODEL FOR EFFECTIVE RETURN-TO-WORK PLANNING

From the University of Cincinnati,
Cincinnati, Ohio

Reprint requests to:
Donald E. Shrey, PhD, CRC
Advanced Transitions, Inc.
2959 Perthwood Drive
Cincinnati, OH 45244

The growth of worksite-based disability management programs represents a major paradigm shift from traditional rehabilitation interventions that focus on the individual, to more holistic, interdisciplinary approaches that address both worksite (environmental) variables and worker (individual) factors.[16] The purpose of this chapter is to provide an overview of the disability management model of work injury management. This model represents a worksite-based approach to early intervention, the goals of which include prevention of chronic and progressive disability, effective return-to-work outcomes, and employment retention of workers with disabilities.

THE DISABILITY MANAGEMENT MODEL: AN OVERVIEW

The disability management model may be best understood in the context of interventions that occur on a continuum, from the point of injury or disability onset, through "job retention" interventions that ensure that the worker has been properly accommodated and that future lost time and work disability will be minimized. Early intervention plus timely return to work is critical to achieving successful outcomes for the worker *and* the employer. Offering workers with restrictions modified work options or transitional work programs is a significant factor in return-to-work outcomes. Formal return-to-work programs have demonstrated recurrent savings for worksites over the past several years. For example, a study compared outcomes from two hospitals, one with a formal return-to-work program and one with no formal program. The hospital with the formal program experienced a 50% decrease in numbers of injuries, while the other hospital's injury rate escalated. Fewer than average lost workdays due to injury were recorded in the hospital with the return-to-work program (13.5 days versus 18.5 days). The workers' compensation experience modification rate (a measure of percentage change in premiums paid to an insurance carrier based on frequency, magnitude, and duration of injury or illness) decreased from 1.35 to 0.86 at the hospital with the formal program. The other hospital's rate increased from 0.63 to 1.08.[5]

The outcomes from several return-to-work programs are documented in the research literature.[15] One model return-to-work program, at TS Trim Industries in Canal Winchester, Ohio, reported exceptionally strong outcomes for its worksite-based disability management program. A consulting physical therapist at the worksite was a key factor in successful return-to-work results. Prior to establishing the program in fiscal year 1994–95, TS Trim had 17 lost-time workers' compensation claims, resulting in 508 total lost days. Medical costs totaled $240,282; wage replacement costs were $144,083. Outcomes reported from June, 1996–May, 1997 were 23 lost-time claims, totaling 311 lost days. Wage replacement costs were reduced to $41,460.

At the Alberni Specialties Division of MacMillan Bloedel, Ltd., in Port Alberni, British Columbia, Canada, the worksite's long-term disability (LTD) and short-term disability (STD) costs were found to be three times the industrial average. A disability management program developed in 1995 achieved a total return of 38 workers over a 2-year period. The average lost time among these workers was 16 months, which is significant in that 1 year or more of lost time typically results in a minimal probability of return to work. LTD premium costs were reduced by 25%; STD premium costs were reduced by 20%; a savings of $1.25 million was realized in one year. [15]

At the Somass Division of MacMillan Bloedel, Ltd., a formal disability management program was initiated as a pilot program to demonstrate the impact of joint labor-management collaboration. Of 120 workers who participated in this program, 112 had returned to work over an 18-month period. Length of lost time ranged from 4 weeks to 13 years. Fourteen workers on LTD returned to work; six of these workers had a total of 148 years of benefits payments remaining, at a net present value of $2.486 million. Workers' compensation costs were reduced by 50%, and the frequency of lost-time accidents was reduced from 48 to 8 incidents. The number of workers on workers' compensation was reduced from 37 in 1991 to five in 1996.[15]

RETURN-TO-WORK PROCESS

Disability management is an interdisciplinary process that requires careful planning, effective coordination, relationship-building, ongoing communication, and the resources of a skilled and knowledgeable return-to-work coordinator. This process involves many steps that parallel the disabled worker's progression from the point of injury or disability through successful return to work. These steps must be orchestrated within the context of disability management policies and procedures that are jointly supported by labor and management. The purpose of the following section is to provide an overview of the steps in the return to work process within a workplace that has developed a strong disability management infrastructure.

It is important to understand that most worksites have fairly standard administrative responses to work-related injuries and nonoccupational illnesses, beginning with the **initial report of an injury or illness.** The failure to complete this first step in a timely fashion may be the initial reason for uncontrolled lost time. Based on audits of thousands of claims files, lag-times between injury occurrence and receipt of first injury report may be as much as 100 days, with 7–10 days lag-time being the norm. Late reporting often results in workers receiving unnecessary medical treatment and lost opportunity for the employer to impact positively on the resolution of disability and early return to work. [3]

It is typically the supervisor who first becomes aware of the initial illness or injury, and it is often the worker's responsibility to promptly report the illness or injury to the immediate supervisor. The supervisor usually is responsible for completing an **accident or illness report,** required by workers' compensation statutes or federal laws dealing with occupational safety and health. Accident and illness incidents may be communicated to others within the workplace, such as safety committees, human resource departments, and insurance managers. Likewise, such incidents may be communicated externally to workers' compensation boards, insurance claims managers or third-party claims administrators, and certain government agencies.

The next step in the process of managing the work injury/illness may be **emergency treatment** or **immediate medical consultation** to evaluate the worker's impairment and to administer immediate treatment. When the injury or illness is expected to result in lost time from work, it is important for the worksite to implement an **early response to expected lost time.** When lost time is anticipated, it is necessary for a designated worksite representative to initiate immediate contact with the worker's treating physician. This is the critical time to communicate to the physician the physical demands of the worker's job, and to ascertain from the physician the worker's restrictions and functional abilities. Such communications between the worksite and the treating physician are often initiated by the worker's supervisor, a representative from a corporate health service (i.e., occupational health nurse, company physician), or a human resource representative. Return-to-work coordinators or designated case managers may also be assigned responsibility at this early phase of the work injury/illness management process. When objective medical evidence suggests that the worker's impairment or illness has resulted in work restrictions that will prevent or delay returning to work, the stage is set for implementing the **return to work plan.**

Steps in the Return-to-Work Plan: An Overview

STEP 1: REFERRAL OF THE WORKER TO THE RETURN-TO-WORK COORDINATOR

Establish Referral Criteria. Policies and procedures must be developed at the worksite to guide the worker and others through the return-to-work process. This process should begin as early as possible after the onset of an injury or disability, and end when the worker has made a safe return to work and evidence suggests that the worker is able to safely perform sustained and productive work activity.

At the beginning of the process, it must be clear who is eligible to participate in the worksite's return-to-work program. Since most workers return to work within a reasonable and expected timeframe following an injury or illness, it is unnecessary for all workers with injuries or illnesses to become involved in a formal program. For example, workers with minor strains or sprains that heal over a normal timeframe or workers afflicted with the flu would be expected to return to work within a reasonable period of time. Once these "reasonable" timeframes are exceeded, for whatever reasons, it becomes increasingly important to establish interventions that enable to worker to return to work without unnecessary delays. Both labor and management representatives should decide and agree upon the criteria for determining the conditions under which workers can achieve maximum benefit from early intervention and return-to-work planning.

Several studies have identified effective strategies for managing back problems during the subacute phase (4–12 weeks post-injury).[2,11] These strategies include a combination of clinical and occupational treatments, such as intensive physical therapy and occupational ergonomics, which effectively compare an assessment of the individual with the demands of the work environment. Significant reductions in lost time and costs have been associated with strategies that focus on worker–work environment relationships. The conclusions of these studies suggest that workers who fail to recover by 4 weeks post-injury are prime candidates for involvement in a return-to-work program.

Here is a sample list of criteria for defining which workers should be given priority for referral to the return-to-work program:

- Worker has not been working for past 30 days due to injury, illness, or disability
- Worker has recently sustained an injury, illness, or disability that is expected to result in 30 days or more lost time from work
- Worker's job is at risk because he/she is unable to perform essential job functions due to restrictions
- Worker has been working in a "light duty" assignment for more than 60 days and has been unable to return to full-duty status; the worker's abilities and limitations are unknown
- Worker has a lost-time injury and has exceeded the expected period of lost time predicted by his or her treating physician.

Consulting the Worker Prior to Return-to-Work Program Referral. Worksites must decide who is responsible for initiating the referral of workers with disabilities to a designated return-to-work (RTW) coordinator. Referral sources vary considerably among worksites, and individuals making referrals to the RTW coordinator may include any of the following: union representatives, members of the worksite's return-to-work or safety committee, human resource managers, immediate supervisors, concerned coworkers, workers with disabilities (self-referral), worksite medical officers, case managers, and safety officers. Regardless of the referral source, all potential referring agents must understand the criteria for referral that has been established by the worksite. In any event, prior to initiating a referral, it is important to consider the following **pre-referral process:**

1. Explain to the worker the purpose and benefits of the worksite's RTW program
2. Provide the worker with written information about the worksite's RTW program, e.g., a copy of a brochure that describes the process and other features of the program
3. Encourage the worker to contact any member of the RTW committee (if one has been established at the worksite) regarding questions about the program
4. Explain to the worker how final approval will be made for his/her involvement in the program
5. Explain to the worker that, after official approval, he/she will be contacted by the RTW coordinator, who will set up an initial meeting.

Prior to initiating a worker referral, it is also helpful for the referring agent to obtain information regarding the essential functions of the worker's job, the worker's abilities and work restrictions, and prior attempts to accommodate the worker in his or her present job or to place the worker in an alternate job. Any special comments or suggestions to the RTW coordinator that may facilitate the worker's involvement in return-to-work activities would also be recommended at this early stage of the process.

STEP 2: WORK ABILITY EVALUATION

The RTW coordinator initiates a work ability evaluation with the worker as early as possible, to avoid unnecessary delays in the return-to-work process. It is reasonable for the coordinator to begin this process within 3 days of the initial referral for services. The following objectives and activities are addressed by the RTW coordinator:

Building Relationships with Workers with Disabilities.   At the initial meeting with the worker, the RTW coordinator focuses on "relationship-building." The initial meeting should be "worker-focused," providing a forum for the worker to express concerns and needs related to return-to-work goals. Concurrently, the RTW coordinator clearly describes his or her roles, functions, and responsibilities as an advocate for the worker during the return-to-work process. The worker is advised of his or her rights at the initial meeting, and the worker's signed consent is obtained to allow the RTW coordinator access to confidential information that may be relevant to return-to-work planning. The use of interpersonal skills and knowledge of human behavior to support and assist the worker is essential to this process.

Return-to-Work Assessment: Review Occupationally Relevant Information. Given the worker's written consent, the RTW coordinator may review any referral information and supportive medical documentation, including independent medical examination or functional capacity reports (if available), to identify objective opinions of clinical experts regarding the worker's functional abilities and work restrictions. This information is critical when determining the worker's ability to safely perform the essential functions of the job.[1,4,7]

Assessment is an essential part of a comprehensive approach to disability management, and may include functional capacity evaluations and workplace assessments such as job analysis. Information obtained from the RTW assessment enables appropriate selection or modification of duties, development of graded RTW programs, and workplace modifications. The determination of the need for further rehabilitation only occurs *after* the assessment phase of the RTW process and/or exhaustive efforts through worksite disability management or successful rehabilitation in a clinical setting.[8]

During the assessment phase of the return-to-work process, the RTW coordinator obtains vocationally relevant information about the worker's:

- Educational and training background
- Work history and transferable work skills
- Hobbies and typical daily activities
- Social activities and support systems
- Personal perspectives on treatments
- Subjective report of functional capacities
- Current work status and relationship with supervisor
- Accommodation needs.

If necessary, an independent functional capacity evaluation may be scheduled to obtain objective measures of the worker's functional abilities.

STEP 3: REVIEW OF CURRENT WORK STATUS AND RETURN-TO-WORK OPTIONS

The RTW coordinator must initiate contact with the worker's supervisor at the worksite to review the worker's current work status (e.g., lost-time patterns, accommodations made, accommodations requested, return-to-work options that are compatible with the worker's restrictions). This direct contact with the supervisor enables the coordinator to assess potential labor relations problems that may impact adversely on RTW planning. More importantly, the coordinator needs to establish a strong, positive relationship with the supervisor and coworkers, to create a supportive environment for accommodations and RTW processes *within the culture of the work unit.*

STEP 4: RETURN-TO-WORK PLAN DEVELOPMENT

If the work ability evaluation results (completed during Step 2) indicate that the worker is capable of performing work, with or without accommodations, an RTW plan is developed to facilitate the return-to-work or work-retention process. This may require the worker to formally request a **reasonable accommodation** (Table 1). This process was addressed by a study of effective interventions for injured nurses in Manitoba, Canada.[19] The interventions resulted in decreased back injuries and associated lost time and costs. An important conclusion was that employees were the best resource for identifying work modifications to facilitate their safe and timely return to work.

Hierarchy of Return-to-Work Options. Within any given worksite, it is important to establish a hierarchy of RTW options (Table 2). Options that are available at the worksite are listed in descending order of priority, beginning with those that (1) pose minimal return to work barriers, (2) require the fewest disability management interventions, and (3) require the least adjustment to be made by the worker.

For example, the **first priority** is to return the worker to the original job at the original worksite. In some instances, this goal may not be achievable due to the worker's permanent restrictions. Therefore, the **second priority** is to return the worker to the original job at the original worksite (with permanent accommodations). When this goal cannot be achieved after all accommodation options have been explored and exhausted, the **third priority** is to return the worker to a similar job within his or her original department or work unit. Maintaining the worker's employment

TABLE 1. The Accommodation Process

1. Discuss the accommodation with the worker who is requesting it.
2. Determine whether existing policies require documentation on the existence of an impairment, to justify the worker's request for an accommodation.
3. Determine whether accommodations are actually required for safe and efficient job performance.
4. Explore at the worksite if accommodations are physically possible for the worker in this position.
5. Examine whether the accommodations under consideration are the most practical, cost-effective, and reasonable methods available to the worker. Consider the following options:
   a. Jobsite accommodations, including job engineering and technical aids
   b. Provision of auxiliary aids, including desk redesign, talking calculators, telephone adaptations, replacing knobs with handles, using sit/stand options, etc.
   c. Job restructuring, to include reassigning incidental tasks, altering parts of several jobs to form one job, job task exchange, job-sharing
   d. Modified work locations, schedules
   e. Barrier removal, such as architectural, communication, and institutional barriers
   f. Reassignment to a vacant position
6. Consider alternatives to the proposed accommodations (have a back-up plan).
7. Determine any adverse effects the accommodation will have on business operations or work productivity.
8. Determine if the accommodations are financially feasible (determine net costs)
9. Determine if the accommodations pose an undue financial hardship on the employer. Review sources for financial assistance to offset the employer's costs.
10. Determine if the proposed accommodations will remove the task barrier in question.
11. Determine if the worker, with the accommodation, will be able to safely perform the job.
12. Identify any medical and safety implications present in the proposed accommodation.
13. Consult with medical and safety staff regarding any health or safety issues that may be present in performing the job tasks with the proposed accommodations.
14. Determine if any third party review of the accommodation is necessary.
15. Inform management and supervisory staff about the proposed accommodation.
16. Determine if suggestions or assistance from other organizational or community resources are needed to implement the accommodation.
17. Maintain a written record of good faith accommodation effort.
18. Have all parties involved sign the final accommodation plan.
19. If the worker refuses the accommodation, document reasons for refusal.
20. Determine if the worker requesting the accommodation requires training in the use of the accommodation.
21. Determine how and when the outcome of the accommodation will be reviewed and evaluated to confirm its effectiveness.

within his or her original department or work unit prevents the worker from facing unnecessary or challenging adjustments when placed in an unfamiliar work unit. Also, the worker often can retain his or her union affiliation and seniority, and benefit by maintaining familiar work activities and relationships with coworkers, union representatives, and supervisors.

DESIGNING THE TRANSITIONAL WORK PROCESS

Transitional work is a progressive, individualized, time-limited process, focused on returning the worker with restrictions to safe and productive employment. It allows the worker with a disability to gradually transition to a targeted job through participation in any combination of the following interventions or services:

- Physical reconditioning at the worksite or at a fitness facility

TABLE 2. A Typical Hierarchy of Worksite Options, in Descending Order of Priority

---

I. Return to Same Job/Same Employer
    A. Return to same job with no accommodations when the worker has no work restrictions.
    B. Return to same job with temporary accommodations when the worker has restrictions and is unable to perform all essential job functions.

When options A & B are not possible, consider the following transitional work process:

    C. Gradual return to work or transitional work program
        1. Implement worksite accommodations.
        2. Identify alternative productive job tasks to be temporarily assigned to the worker.
        3. Involve the worker in physical reconditioning activities and safe work practice training.
        4. Coordinate periodic onsite assessments of the worker's progress and communicate results to the treating physician.
        5. Gradually increase the worker's hours and/or increase the worker's involvement in performing increasingly demanding job tasks.
        6. Consult with the treating physician to eliminate the worker's restrictions, based on the worker's progress, adaptation to job demands, and work performance.
        7. Complete the worker's transition to the original job as the worker's functional abilities become compatible with the essential job tasks of the original job.

If the worker is unable to achieve a successful transition to the original job, consider the following options:

    D. Return to different (modified) job/same employer (whenever possible, review RTW options within the worker's original work unit; consider the worker's transferable work skills and qualifications, as well as any risks or safety issues.)
    E. Provide on-the-job training for the worker to obtain qualifications for performing an alternate job with the original employer.

If all return-to-work options with the original employer have been exhausted, consider the following options:

II. Return to Work with Different Employer
    A. Return to similar job (consider transferable work skills to perform a similar job that is within the worker's functional abilities).
    B. Return to different (or modified) job.
    C. Obtain training through vocational rehabilitation services to gain qualifications for a job.

If return-to-work options with a different employer have been exhausted, consider the following options:

III. Training for Self-Employment
    A. Refer the worker to vocational assessment services to determine potential for benefiting from training for self-employment.
    B. Review the marketability of skills acquired by the worker.

- Job modification
- Safe work practices training
- Assignment to meaningful, alternate, productive job tasks (which may be identified through the development of a job bank) or to a cluster of work-related activities that require low physical demands, to extend options for temporary transitional work assignments
- Development of individualized transitional work plans (including consultation with worksite managers, supervisors, case managers, treating physicians, other treatment providers, and external resources.

The scientific literature on modified work and RTW programs has been systematically reviewed to assess the effectiveness of these programs.[9] The main finding was that modified work programs facilitate return to work for temporarily and permanently disabled workers. The analysis of 13 high-quality studies suggested that those workers who are offered modified work options return to work about twice as often as those who are not offered such RTW opportunities. These researchers also found that modified work programs cut the number of lost work days in half, with evidence suggesting that modified work programs are cost-effective.

Individualized transitional work plans are developed concurrently with an assessment of the worker's functional abilities, as relates to the physical demands of the job. Workers requiring more than basic accommodations may benefit from involvement in a transitional work program. The worker's transitional work plan is a written document, designed with the worker's active involvement, to identify specific tasks to be performed for designated time periods. Worker participation in conditioning activities may be combined with work activities for optimal strengthening and safe work performance. Jobsite modifications and accommodations are also important components of a transitional work plan, ensuring greater compatibility between physical job demands and the worker's functional capacities.

The success of a transitional work plan is only limited by the flexibility and creativity of those involved in developing it. Transitional work is defined as: **any combination of tasks, functions, jobs or therapeutic activities that a worker with functional restrictions can perform safely, for pay, and without the risk of injury to self or other workers.** Transitional work is typically limited to 8–12 weeks maximum duration. The transitional work process includes ongoing evaluation of the worker's job performance, with gradual upgrading of job tasks as the worker gains strength and endurance through proper exercise, therapy, and conditioning activities.

After the worker begins the transitional work process, ongoing monitoring of the worker's progress is performed by the supervisor or other designated worksite representative. In some worksites, physical therapists, occupational therapists, exercise physiologists, or occupational health nurses may perform periodic monitoring of workers to document progress. As the worker progresses through conditioning and work readjustment, the more physically challenging job tasks are introduced to the worker's daily work assignments, with more of the worker's original job tasks gradually reassigned. Workers who begin transitional work on a part-time basis may also have their work hours or workdays gradually increased, as they achieve higher levels of safe work performance. Worker monitoring, when done in a caring fashion, gives assurance that both labor and management value the injured worker as a contributing member of the work group.

Creating Return-To-Work Options

There are multiple strategies to create RTW options for workers with restrictions. Work tasks in the worker's original job can be modified or temporarily assigned to other workers, as an accommodation strategy. Workers with restrictions can be offered a **gradual return to work** option, which involves the gradual increase of time spent performing the job as the worker's strength and endurance increases. Less demanding tasks of the worker's original job can be combined with temporarily assigned job tasks that are compatible with the worker's abilities. These newly assigned job tasks can be gradually changed to more physically challenging tasks, as the worker's strength and endurance increases. The worker may temporarily be assigned to an alternate job within the same department or work unit or within a different department, followed by a gradual transition to the original job. Worksites can create temporary job assignments that are not part of existing jobs, but which may be meaningful and productive and may contribute to the work processes of others (e.g., recylcing, filing, customer service telephone calls, safety inspections, inventory work, training). Worksites can create a formal job bank, which serves as a reservoir of job tasks that can be temporarily assigned to the worker while he or she is recovering from an injury or illness.

Job Banks

Transitional work programs are often strengthened by developing a job bank, which is a cluster of temporary, meaningful, and productive jobs or job tasks (sedentary to light work activity) that can be performed while the worker is making a recovery from the injury or illness. Work tasks and jobs from the job bank can be flexibly assigned to workers, on a day-to-day basis, to facilitate a return to the worker's regular job or to a permanent modified job. For example, if the worker is unable to perform the essential functions of his or her regular job, then only those original job tasks that are compatible with his/her functional capacities are part of the modified job. The job bank is an effective resource that helps to reduce or eliminate lost time, which relates directly to reduced worker's compensation and other disability costs (Table 3).

TABLE 3. A Typical Method for Creating a Job Bank

1. Observe the actual job task(s) while it is performed in the normal work environment.
2. If the worker is restricted in the ability to perform a specific task, such as extended standing, the job analysis may focus on that one physical ability.
3. Identify each of the major job tasks, using "job task statements" that begin with action verbs, such as:
   • Lifts boxes of paper to the sorting table
   • Pushes cart with supplies to the mail room
   • Carries files to cabinet for filing
4. Job tasks may be: Physical—operates power drill
                      Mental—analyzes data
                      Interpersonal—trains management team
5. Identify **tools and equipment** that the worker uses to perform the tasks.
6. Indicate the **frequency** or time required for the worker to perform a specific job task:
   • The worker stands up to 30 minutes on a continuous basis two times during the 8-hour shift.
   • Average lifting is in the 5 lb. range or less on an intermittent basis throughout the work shift. Maximum lifting is 25 lbs. which is performed once per shift.
   Establish detailed and concise information on tasks in the job bank, since this information will be compared with the worker's functional abilities to perform these tasks when involved in transitional work.
7. Identify hazards or risk factors associated with the job tasks that may cause reinjury or an aggravation of the worker's disability (e.g., mechanical, electrical, moving objects, dangerous equipment, sharp tools, slippery floors, unprotected heights).
8. For each task in the job bank, create a standard form to record information that classifies the task according to:
   • Name of department or work unit
   • Time required to complete task
   • Description of job site
   • Tools and equipment used
   • Physical requirements to perform task
   • Exertional level of task
   • Hazards or risks and injury prevention controls

Job banks can be created within a work unit or within an entire workplace by identifying and classifying tasks that can be performed safely by workers with restrictions. Job tasks may last only 1 hour or they may be combined to last a full 8-hour workday. Job banks are typically comprised of job tasks or work activities that do not exceed 20 lbs. of lifting and carrying, and they generally do not involve excessive or repetitive postural changes (e.g., constant or continuous bending, stooping, above-shoulder reaching, pushing/pulling, crawling). Job bank tasks often include work activities that can be performed while seated or tasks that allow the worker to alternate sitting and standing.

Safe Work Practices: Training and Physical Conditioning

Workers involved in transitional work programs may concurrently participate in safe work practices education and training and physical conditioning to increase strength and endurance. Such training and conditioning is often provided by occupational therapists, physical therapists, and exercise physiologists, who are familiar with body mechanics and physiology related to work. They train workers on job risks and safety precautions, such as lifting techniques, body mechanics, and working postures for sitting, reaching, standing, bending, and twisting. They teach workers proper exercise techniques to strengthen muscles and to increase flexibility and endurance. An overview of this process is offered in *Sourcebook of Occupational Rehabilitation.*[10]

> *Strengthening exercises to condition the muscles that will be used to perform the job activity and endurance training exercises that will allow the individual to withstand the particular physical stresses on the job are crucial to injury prevention. An example of how these components can be implemented is as follows: An individual works on a loading dock. He or she performs activities that require lifting, pushing, and pulling objects (based on a job analysis). At times, he or she must be able to move quickly along the dock as the merchandise arrives. To prevent injuries, the subject should be trained in proper lifting techniques (education and training); regularly perform exercises to strengthen the abdominals, quadriceps, and lower spine; and perform aerobic exercises, such as walking or running. (p. 137)*

Identifying Transferable Skills

During the assessment phase of the return to work process, the RTW coordinator obtains information from the worker and the worksite about skills and occupationally relevant qualifications the worker may have acquired through education or training, or through the performance of work activities. Occupations are generally classified as unskilled, semi-skilled, and skilled.

Unskilled work is work that requires little or no judgment to do simple duties that can be learned on the job in a short period of time. The job may or may not require considerable strength. For example, jobs may be considered unskilled if the primary work duties are handling, feeding and offbearing (that is, placing or removing materials from machines that are automatic or operated by others), or machine tending; a person can usually learn to do the job in 30 days or less; and little specific vocational preparation and judgment are needed. A worker does not gain work skills by performing unskilled jobs.

Semi-skilled work is work that requires some skills, but does not require doing the more complex work duties. Semi-skilled jobs may require alertness and close attention to watching machine processes; inspecting, testing, or otherwise looking for irregularities; tending or guarding equipment, property, materials, or persons against loss, damage, or injury; or other types of activities that are similarly less complex than skilled work, but more complex than unskilled work. A job may be classified as semi-skilled if coordination and dexterity are necessary, as when hands or feet must be moved quickly to do repetitive tasks.

Skilled work requires the worker to use judgment to determine the machine and manual operations to be performed to obtain the proper form, quality, or quantity of material to be produced. Skilled work may require laying out work, estimating quality, determining the suitability and needed quantities of materials, making precise measurements, reading blueprints or other specifications, or making computations or mechanical adjustments to control or regulate the work. Other skilled jobs may require dealing with people, facts or figures, or abstract ideas at a high level of complexity.

"Transferability" refers to skills that can be used in other work. This is important in the context of disability management, since workers with disabilities sometimes have permanent work restrictions that prevent them from returning to their original jobs. The results of a "transferability of skills analysis" may establish the worker's qualifications to perform other work that is compatible with the worker's functional abilities.

A worker has skills that can be used in other jobs when the skilled or semi-skilled work activities that he or she did in the past can be used to meet the requirements of skilled or semi-skilled work activities of other jobs or other kinds of work. This depends largely on the similarity of occupationally significant work activities among different jobs. Transferability is most probable and meaningful among jobs in which:

- The same or a lesser degree of skill is required;
- The same or similar tools and machines are used; and
- The same or similar raw materials, products, processes, or services are involved.

There are degrees of transferability of skills ranging from very close similarities to remote and incidental similarities among jobs. A complete similarity of all three factors above is not necessary for transferability. However, when skills are so specialized or have been acquired in such an isolated vocational setting (like many jobs in mining, agriculture, or fishing) that they are not readily usable in other industries, jobs, and work settings, they are not considered transferable.

FACTORS THAT IMPACT THE RETURN TO WORK

The factors related to return to work after illness or injury have been reported by several researchers.[6,12,13,14,17,18] There is no consistent evidence to suggest which particular factors are associated with successful RTW outcomes. Research studies on RTW factors vary considerably, based on diagnoses, types of injuries, severity of disability, and how "successful outcome" is defined. The factors related to return to work often include age, gender, educational level, marital status, severity of illness or injuries, injury to admission time, and job attachment to the pre-injury employer. Worksite variables, however, have been given relatively little notice among researchers. This is an area where more research is required, since return to work success is highly dependent upon worksite' readiness to accommodate workers with restrictions. In turn, the worksite's capacity to accommodate workers with restrictions is strongly related to supportive policies, procedures, and other worksite-specific factors.

Overall, successful RTW outcomes can be affected by factors specific to: (1) the worker with a disability, (2) the work environment, (3) the availability and quality of community resources and services, and (4) laws and regulations related to employer obligations, workers' compensation statutes, disability insurance policies, and government programs. More research is needed to investigate how these multiple factors interact to support RTW outcomes for persons with disabilities.

Factors specific to the worker with a disability

- Job satisfaction
- Motivation to return to work
- Economic incentives/disincentives to work

- Psychosocial readiness to return to work
- Physical abilities
- Psychological abilities
- Transferable work skills and work qualifications
- Age and educational/training background
- Family supports
- Level of medical improvement of worker's impairment

Factors specific to the work environment
- Joint labor-management support for worksite RTW program
- Accountability and authority among worksite representatives who are responsible for implementing RTW activities
- Corporate culture — worker and supervisor expectations regarding RTW processes and activities
- Internal communications at the worksite during the RTW coordination process
- External communications — between the worksite and community rehabilitation providers, treating physicians, insurance claims representatives, case managers, and others
- Benefit plan design and influences — disability insurance policies that promote and reward RTW activities versus prolonged and unmanaged disability
- Knowledge and skills of RTW coordinator
- Accident prevention and safety programs
- Occupational ergonomics
- Health promotion and wellness programs
- Early intervention and worker monitoring protocol
- Case management procedures
- Return-to-work coordination
- Transitional work options
- Worksite accommodations

Factors specific to the availability and quality of community resources and services
- Medical specialty services (i.e., orthopedics, neurology, occupational medicine, psychiatry, pain clinics)
- Physical conditioning services — occupational therapists, physical therapists, exercise physiologists
- Psychological and behavioral medicine services
- Occupational ergonomics and rehabilitation engineering
- Case management/medical management services
- Alcohol and substance abuse treatment facilities
- Disability-specific resources (e.g., Multiple Sclerosis Society, services for visually impaired persons, cardiac rehabilitation services, head injury treatment programs, orthotic and prosthetic services)
- Vocational rehabilitation services (e.g., vocational evaluation centers, work adjustment services, career counseling services, job placement services)
- Transitional work/disability management technical assistance services
- Health promotion, injury prevention, and safety services

Factors specific to laws and regulations
- Workers' compensation statutes that promote RTW services and programs
- Industrial hygiene and safety resources available through insurance policies
- Claims management procedures provided by workers' compensation boards and private disability insurance companies
- Americans with Disabilities Act

- Government services and incentive programs related to reintegration of persons with disabilities

The disability management model, as outlined in this chapter, represents an approach to achieving successful return-to-work outcomes. This model, which has been successfully demonstrated among pro-active worksites, addresses many of the above factors through a coordinated process. Building a strong worksite infrastructure to support RTW activities is the key to protecting the employability of workers with disabilities. Worksite-based disability management programs, when fully supported by labor and management, result in recurrent savings to employers. Formal RTW programs that are strengthened by effective policies and operational procedures, and linked with responsive rehabilitation resources, also result in safe and sustained employment for persons with disabilities.

REFERENCES

1. Alexander J, Fuhrer, M: Functional assessment of individuals with physical impairments. In Harlpern, A, Fuhrer, M (eds): Functional Assessment in Rehabilitation. Baltimore, MD, Paul H. Brookes, 1984, pp 45–59.
2. Brooker A, Clarke J, Sinclair S et al: Effective Disability Management and Return to Work Practices. Paper Presented at National Leadership Roundtable on Employee Health by Institute for Work and Health, Toronto, April 28–29, 1998.
3. Douglas J: Managing Workers' Compensation: A Human Resources Guide to Controlling Costs. New York, NY, Wiley & Sons, 1994.
4. Fraser T: Fitness for Work: The Role of Physical Demands Analysis and Physical Capacity Assessment. Bristol, PA, Taylor and Francis, 1992.
5. Gice J, Tompkins K: Return to work program in a hospital setting. J Bus Psychol 4 (2):237–243, 1989.
6. Graly J, Jensen G, Gibson M, Laborde T: Factors influencing return to work for clients in a work-hardening center. Work 4:9–21, 1994.
7. Hart D, Isernhagen S, Matheson L: Guidelines for functional capacity evaluation of people with medical conditions. J Orthoped Sports Phys Ther 18:682–686, 1993.
8. Innes E, Straker L: A clinician's guide to work-related assessments: I. Purposes and problems. Work 11:183–189, 1998.
9. Karuse N, Dasinger L, Neuhaser F: Modified work and return to work: A review of the literature. J Occup Rehabil 8 (2):113–139, 1998.
10. King P (ed): Concepts and Practices of Occupational Rehabilitation. New York, NY, Plenum, 1998.
11. Lindstrom I, Ohlund C, Eek E, et al: The effect of graded activity on patients with subacute low back pain: A randomized prospective clinical study with an operant-conditioning behavioural approach. Phys Ther 72 (4):279–293, 1992.
12. Moffroid M, Aja D, Haugh L, Henry S: Efficacy of a part-time work hardening program for persons with low-back pain. Work 3: 14–20, 1993.
13. Niemeyer L, Jacobs K, Reynolds-Lynch K, et al: Work hardening: Past, present, and future—the work programs special interest section national work-hardening outcome study. Am J Occup Ther 48:327–339, 1994.
14. Schmidt S, Oort-Marburger D, Meijman T: Employment after rehabilitation for musculoskeletal impairments: The impact of vocational rehabilitation and working on a trial basis. Arch Phys Med Rehabil 76:950–954, 1995.
15. Shrey D: Effective worksite-based disability management programs. In King, P (ed): Concepts and Practices of Occupational Rehabilitation. New York, NY, Plenum, 1998, pp 389–409.
16. Shrey D: Disability management in industry: The new paradigm in injured worker rehabilitation. Disabil Rehabil 18 (8):408–414, 1996.
17. Tate D: Workers disability and return to work. Am J Phys Med Rehabil 71:92–96, 1992.
18. Voaklander D, Beaulne A, Lessard R:.Factors related to outcome following a work hardening program. J Occup Rehabil 5:71–85, 1995.
19. Yassi A: Early intervention for back-injured nurses at a large Canadian tertiary care hospital: An evaluation of the effectiveness and cost benefit of a two-year pilot project. Occup Med 45 (4):209–214, 1995.

TIMOTHY PROCTOR, PhD CANDIDATE
ROBERT J. GATCHEL, PhD
RICHARD C. ROBINSON, PhD

PSYCHOSOCIAL FACTORS AND RISK OF PAIN AND DISABILITY

From The University of Texas
   Southwestern Medical Center
Dallas, Texas

Reprint requests to:
Timothy Proctor, PhD Cand.
Department of Psychiatry
University of Texas Southwestern
   Medical Center
5323 Harry Hines Blvd.
Dallas, TX 75235-9044

This research was supported in
part by grants to Dr. Gatchel from
the National Institutes of Health
(2R01 MH46452 and R01
DE10713).

The cost of chronic pain, in terms of personal suffering and financial impact, is staggering. Approximately 70–80% of adults develop a spinal disorder during their life.[15,37] Fortunately, 90% of spinal disorders resolve within 6 months. However, the remaining 10% who develop chronic pain and disability account for the majority of the expenses.[2] It has been estimated that 15% of adults are totally and permanently disabled by chronic spinal disorders;[26] that $16 billion is spent annually on spinal pain patients;[32] and that $27 billion is spent on all musculoskeletal patients.[26] In fact, when all treatment costs are included (e.g., social security, lost productivity), the annual cost is estimated at $20 to 60 billion.[41]

Complicating a difficult problem is the common clinical observation that patients with chronic pain disorders present with concurrent psychiatric disorders that contribute to their pain, suffering, and disability. For instance, one study reported that chronic low back pain (LBP) patients experience more depression and have higher rates of substance abuse and personality disorders than the general population.[36]

PSYCHOSOCIAL ASPECTS OF CHRONIC PAIN

Research over the past three decades has clearly demonstrated the central importance of psychosocial factors in the perception and reporting of chronic pain and disability.[22,23,35,51,44] As early as 1959, Engel[17] argued that the perception of pain is a psychological phenomenon. He also described personality characteristics that he hypothesized predisposed individuals to chronic pain. These characteristics included a history of defeat, significant guilt, unsatisfied aggressive impulses, and a propensity to develop pain in response to a real or imagined loss. Gatchel and Epker[25] have provided an updated review of many of the psychosocial risk factors.

Melzack and Wall's[43] **gate control theory of pain** represented an important milestone by hypothesizing that central nervous system mechanisms provided the physiological basis for psychological involvement in pain perception. Specifically, these researchers theorized that a neurophysiological mechanism in the spinal cord, located in the dorsal horns, acted as a gate for pain signals and allowed for modulation from various sources. Thus, the gate control theory integrated peripheral stimuli with cortical variables, explaining the impact that mood states may have on pain perception.

The **biopsychosocial model** combined social factors with the psychological and physiological components of pain. Turk and Rudy[56] elaborated and refined Melzak and Wall's[43] early assumptions by incorporating cognitive, affective, psychosocial, behavioral, and physiological elements into the chronic pain experience. Their research suggested that, as suffering increases, psychosocial factors play an increasingly significant role in the perpetuation of pain behavior and suffering.

Psychopathology and Chronic LBP

The central importance of psychosocial factors in the pain perception process has come to be accepted by the scientific community. The majority of the research conducted in this area has focused on the relationship between pain and depression. Several studies have reported extremely high rates of major depressive disorder in chronic pain patients, with current and lifetime rates of rates of 45% and 65%, respectively, in the chronic LBP population, and both current and lifetime rates of about 80% in the chronic upper extremity population.[36,44] Note, however, that the reported prevalence rates of depression in chronic pain patients vary a great deal. In fact, prevalence rates of 31–100% have been reported.[46] Most studies report prevalence rates that can be classified in the moderately high range. For instance, a recent study conducted by Banks and Kerns[4] addressed this issue through a review of 14 studies that utilized the *Diagnostic and Statistical Manual* (DSM) criteria for diagnosing major depression in chronic pain patients. The authors reported that 9 of the 14 studies reviewed reported prevalence rates of major depression in chronic pain patients to be 30–54%. These percentages can be compared with recent estimates of current and lifetime major depression for the entire United States population, which are 5% and 17%, respectively.[9]

Another group[19] reported a number of interesting findings after exploring this relationship via a meta-analysis of studies that concerned both chronic pain and depression. Of the 23 studies reviewed, 21 related the *severity* of pain to the degree of depression. Each of the three studies reviewed that focused on the association between pain *duration* and the development of depression found a relationship between these two variables. In addition, a relationship was found between pain *frequency* and depression in all four of the reviewed studies that focused on this connection. The authors examined two studies that looked at the association between depression and the *number of pain sites*. Both of these studies reported a relationship between the two variables, with multiple-site pain patients being much more likely to be depressed than single-site pain patients.

Demographic and work-related variables that impact the risk of disability due to the combination of depression and chronic pain has also been explored in the literature with mixed findings.[3] A study by Averill and colleagues[3] provided some clarity to this issue with a group of 254 chronic pain patients. In addition to addressing pain-related variables, the authors conducted a comprehensive examination of a number of demographic and work-related variables. Overall, the variable of **work status** (employment) was the most highly related to increased depression in chronic pain patients, followed by education level and martial status. The strong relationship between work status and depression in chronic pain patients is consistent with an earlier study by Magni and colleagues[38] in which unemployment was associated with increased levels of depression. With respect to **education level,** lower levels of education related to increased depressive symptoms in chronic pain patients. The authors postulate that this finding may be the result of the fewer alternative work options that are available to those with lower education levels. Reasoning skills that are more concrete in nature, and less flexibility in coping options, are also proposed as possible explanations. As for **marital status,** single status was found to be highly related to increased levels of depression. This finding is in contrast to an earlier study[30] that found no relation between depression and marital status in chronic pain patients.

In addition to the three variables that accounted for the majority of the variance (work status, education level, and marital status), an interaction was found between depression and several other variables. With respect to demographic variables, age and gender interacted with depression, with younger women endorsing more depressive symptomatology than younger men, and older men scoring higher than older women. No relation was found between ethnicity and depression among the chronic pain patients. As for work-related variables, a significant interaction was found between planned litigation and work status, which is consistent with other results.[53] Chronic pain patients who were working and planning litigation had higher levels of depression than patients who were working and not planning litigation; patients who were both not working and not planning litigation were more depressed than those who were not working, but were planning litigation. In explaining these findings, the authors postulate that depression in individuals that are both working and litigating may be the result of an "internal conflict" about their two contradictory roles. As for those who are neither working nor litigating, the authors suggest that feelings of powerlessness and hopelessness may be responsible for their depressive symptomatology.

A number of studies have looked at the way in which co-occurrence of depression and chronic pain impacts treatment and subsequent disability. One group[59] found that chronic LBP patients with depression avoid activities more than those who do not suffer from depression. The authors also reported that depressed patients engage in more self-blame and display a greater tendency to avoid social support and behaviors aimed at problem solving. Dworkin and colleagues[16] looked at a group of chronic pain patients and determined that those suffering from depression were less likely to benefit from treatment. Haley and associates[29] reported that chronic pain patients treated with antidepressant medications reported less pain-related symptoms, while Von Korff and Simon[58] found that patients' depressive symptoms improve when their pain symptoms are alleviated. In addition to these findings, it has also been noted that depressed patients magnify the perception of pain and have a lower pain tolerance.[3]

In summary, it is clear that a relationship exists between depression and chronic pain. The degree of depression is related to the presence, frequency, duration, and severity of pain. There is also a strong relationship between depression and the number of pain sites. Depressed chronic pain patients tend to magnify their symptoms, avoid more activities, benefit less from treatment, and engage in more self-blaming behaviors. Work status, level of education, and marital status appear to be the most important correlates of depression in chronic pain population. In addition to these three variables, a number of other demographic, pain-related, and work-related variables appear to be associated with depression in the chronic pain population. This information is of use because it can aid in predicting pain patients who are at risk of becoming depressed and increasingly disabled due to the combination of depression and chronic pain. With these patients, early preventative treatments may decrease the likelihood of long-term disability.

The Relationship Between Pain and Psychopathology

It is evident that chronic pain is a complex psychophysiological behavior pattern that is not amenable to simple component analyses of psychological, social, and physical factors. One of the more vexing questions about the relationship between pain and psychopathology involves the question, "Which comes first: the pain or the psychopathology?" This question does not have a simple answer, but researchers are beginning to develop a better understanding of the relationship between pain and psychopathology.

Several studies have provided evidence that chronic pain clearly contributes to the expression of psychological distress and psychopathology. Sternbach and associates [51] compared the Minnesota Multiphasic Personality Inventory (MMPI) profiles of acute and chronic pain patients and found that the chronic pain patients reported significantly more psychological distress as measured by the first three clinical scales of the MMPI (scale 1—hypochondriasis; scale 2—depression; and scale 3—hysteria; also known as "the neurotic triad"). Barnes and colleagues[5] obtained similar results with the MMPI, finding that 6 months after successfully completing an intensive 3-week rehabilitation program, when a majority of the patients had returned to work, previously elevated measures of distress had returned to normal levels.

Another group[44] also attempted to delineate the complex relationship between psychopathology and pain. Using the Structured Clinical Interview for the *DSM of Mental Disorders-III-Revised,* they found that of 200 chronic LBP patients, 77% met lifetime diagnostic criteria for psychiatric disturbances. The most common diagnoses were depression, substance abuse, and anxiety disorders. In addition, 51% of the patients met criteria for a personality disorder. In an examination of 152 chronic LBP patients prior to undergoing an intensive 3-week functional restoration program, it was found that 90% of the chronic LBP patients met criteria for a lifetime axis I diagnosis; the most prevalent diagnoses were major depression and substance abuse.[27]

Although more prospective studies need to be conducted to examine the extent to which psychopathology predisposes an individual to pain, research into personality disorders provides us with clues. Personality disorders are defined by the DSM-IV as life-long maladaptive patterns of perceiving, relating to, and thinking about the environment and oneself, that are exhibited in a wide range of social and personal contexts.[1] According to this definition, personality disorders cannot result from the stress associated with dealing with chronic pain. Fishbain and colleagues[20] found an incidence of 58.4% of axis II disorders in chronic LBP patients. Other researchers have found similar incidence rates of axis II pathology, which are at or above 50% for chronic LBP populations, far above the percentage found in the general population.[27,45]

Research investigating childhood abuse and pain also provides us with information about the ways disruptive developmental experiences impact personality, psychopathology, and pain. As early as 1859, Briquet in his *Traite de l'hysterie* believed there to be a relationship between childhood abuse and somatoform disorders (as cited in Mai and Merskey[39]). Since that time, several studies have demonstrated an association between pain and abuse.[6,31,10]

Schofferman and associates[48] investigated spinal surgery outcomes and psychosocial risk factors, including physical abuse, sexual abuse, substance abuse by caregivers, abandonment, and emotional neglect. As expected, most of the patients who denied all of these risk factors had positive outcomes, but significantly fewer patients who reported three or more of these risk factors had positive outcomes. Essentially the same group of investigators also found a high correlation between childhood trauma and chronic LBP.[49] These findings are consistent with another study,42 in which investigators found that female chronic LBP patients had a higher rate of childhood abuse than a control group without a history of chronic pain. Further, chronic LBP patients with a history of childhood abuse had more lifetime axis I diagnoses, more lifetime axis II diagnoses, a lower return-to-work rate, and a higher number of post-discharges.[42]

Gatchel[24] attempted to clarify this complex relationship between pain, psychopathology, and personality by theorizing about the progression from of acute to chronic pain. He refers to the psychological changes that occur as a person progresses from acute to chronic pain as a "layering of behavioral/psychological problems over the original nociception of the pain experience itself." His model is based on a **three-stage progression** from acute to subacute to chronic disability, following the experience of pain as a result of an identifiable injury. Stage 1 encompasses the resulting emotional reactions (e.g., fear, anxiety, and worry) which arise as a consequence of perceived pain. Stage 2 begins when the pain persists past a reasonable, acute time period. It is at this stage that the development or exacerbation of psychological and behavioral problems occurs. Gatchel notes that the form these difficulties take depends primarily on the premorbid personality and psychological characteristics of the individual (i.e., a diathesis), as well as current socioeconomic and environmental stressors. For instance, an individual with a tendency to become depressed may develop a depressive disorder in response to the economic and social stress of being unable to work as a result of pain.[28] Such a **diathesis-stress model** has also been recently amplified by Weisberg and colleagues.[60]

This complex interaction of physical and psychosocioeconomic factors leads to Stage 3 of the model. As the patient's life begins to totally and completely revolve around the pain as a result of the chronic nature of the problem, he or she begins to accept the sick role. By doing so, the patient is excused from normal responsibilities and social obligations, and such avoidance may serve to reinforce the maintenance of the sick role.

Further adding to the "layers" of behavioral and psychosocial difficulties is the addition of physical deconditioning, which generally accompanies patients during their progression toward chronic disability. The **physical deconditioning** syndrome leads to the progressive lack of use of the body, as when an individual is physically and emotionally distressed. Research has shown that this physical deconditioning can produce a circular effect, leading to increased mental deconditioning. The combined interaction of the symptoms as they reinforce one another negatively impacts the emotional well-being and self-esteem of an individual.[28] Conversely, these same negative emotional reactions can reinforce the physical deconditioning through decreased motivation to participate in work and recreational activities. Further complicating the process, when patients engage in an activity that produces acute pain, they are likely to associate the pain with the initial hurt. This causes patients to fear and avoid pain and possible pain-producing situations. Unfortunately, pain often accompanies physical reconditioning and the additional steps needed to resume normal responsibilities and social obligations. Therefore, patients must be taught that *hurt and harm are not the same.*[23]

COPING

The ways an individual manages and copes with general stressors, and the multifaceted stress of chronic pain, have been implicated as important in relationship to emotional distress, psychopathology, and predicting who will become chronic. The Multidimensional Pain Inventory (MPI)[35], formerly the West-Haven Yale Multidimensional Pain Inventory, is one of the most widely used measures in the pain area. The MPI is a brief, self-report instrument that examines the person's perception of pain and coping ability.

The MPI helps to identify patients having difficulty coping with their pain and can guide the implementation of pain reduction interventions. Turk and Rudy[54] identified three coping styles using a cluster analysis on the MPI scales with a heterogeneous group of chronic pain patients: dysfunctional (43%), interpersonally distressed (28%), and adaptive copers (29.5%). The **dysfunctional** group members reported that their pain, and the interference caused by their pain, was extreme. Patients in the **interpersonally distressed** group reported a lack of support, caring, and understanding from their family members and significant others. In contrast, individuals in the **adaptive copers** group reported high levels of activity and life control as well as lower levels of pain intensity, perceived interference, and affective distress.

The MPI has become well established as a useful tool in the assessment of patients with chronic pain conditions such as low back pain, cancer, fibromyalgia, and temporomandibular disorders.[55] For example, in a recent study by Epker and Gatchel[18] it was found that a group of temporomandibular patients with either dysfunctional or interpersonally distressed profiles on the MPI, demonstrated more acute and chronic biopsychosocial difficulties than patients with adaptive coper profiles.

Brown and Nicassio[11] have described adaptive coping strategies that are similar to the activities of adaptive copers on the MPI. These investigators noted an association between reduction in pain perception and active coping strategies such as staying busy, distraction techniques, and ignoring the pain. In contrast, more passive strategies, such as limiting one's activities and wishful thinking, appear associated with more severe pain. These studies highlight the importance of coping, both in relation to pain and psychopathology.

CATASTROPHIZING

The role of catastrophizing in the prediction of chronic pain and disability has gained increased attention in recent years. Catastrophizing involves thinking negatively, and in an exaggerated fashion, about events and stimuli. This can be applied to how a person perceives his or her pain or the person's ability to cope with the pain.[52] One of the first studies to address this variable[12] looked at cognitive strategies and postoperative pain in a sample of general surgical patients. Investigators found that increased catastrophizing was associated with higher levels of postoperative pain intensity. Main and Waddell[40] also looked at this variable and found a strong relationship between catastrophizing and depressive symptoms in a sample of LBP patients. Further, of the cognitive variables investigated by the authors, catastrophizing was determined to have the "greatest potential for understanding current low back symptoms."[40] Jacobsen and Butler[33] examined the role of catastrophizing in 59 females who had undergone surgery for breast cancer and found that increased catastrophizing was associated with more intense pain and greater use of analgesic medications. In addition, age was determined to be an important predictor of catastrophizing and postoperative pain, with younger patients being more likely to catastrophize and endorse greater levels of pain. A study by Sullivan and colleagues[52] investigated the function of catastrophizing in the prediction of pain and disability in sample of 86 patients with various types of soft-tissue injuries. In this study, catastrophizing was associated with perceived disability, reported pain intensity, and employment status. In addition, catastrophizing "contributed to the prediction of disability over and above the variance accounted for by pain intensity" and was related to disability independent of anxiety and depression levels.

Individuals who catastrophize experience increased pain intensity and, in one study, used larger amounts of analgesics. Younger patients appear to possess a greater tendency to catastrophize, which may result in the experience of higher levels of pain. Catastrophizing appears to be an important variable in the prediction of disability following an injury, with one study finding it to be a more powerful predictor than pain intensity. Fortunately, catastrophizing is amenable and especially suited for cognitive-behavioral interventions.

The Influence of Job Satisfaction and Chronic Pain on Disability

Another factor that is associated with chronic pain, and subsequent disability, is job satisfaction. A number of retrospective studies have found an association between pain and job satisfaction,[8] as have several prospective studies.[7,13,14] In each of these studies, decreased job satisfaction was related to increased pain-related symptoms, and in many cases it was also related to increased chronicity.

A recent study by Williams and colleagues[61] investigated the role of job satisfaction in the progression from acute to chronic pain. Specifically, the authors looked at the extent to which job satisfaction predicted disability, pain, and psychological distress 6 months following the onset of low back pain in 82 males. The results of this study indicated that job satisfaction may serve a protective role against the development of chronic pain and disability following an initial acute onset of back pain. These findings also revealed that dissatisfaction with one's job may increase the risk of long-term disability.

Vingard and colleagues[57] addressed the association between job satisfaction and pain-related disability in a sample of 2118 males and females. In contrast to earlier studies,[7,14] the results of this investigation indicated that job dissatisfaction increased the risk of low back pain in males, but not in females. In addition, an increased risk of low back pain was seen in men who reported "mostly routine work and no possibilities for learning;" however, this was also not the case in females.[57] As a possible explanation of these findings, the authors proposed that females might be more satisfied with their work situations or have lower overall job expectations than men. Although previous studies have found an association between job satisfaction and pain in both males and females, this study raises the possibility that this association may differ by gender. However, additional research is necessary to more fully explore this possibility.

CONCLUSION

An appropriate conclusion of this article is to cite Sanders,[47] who recently provided a brief overview of risk factors that appear to predict the occurrence of low back pain and the development of chronic disability (defined as pain disability lasting 3 months or more). The majority of these 11 factors are psychosocial, behavioral, or environmental in nature (Table 1).

As Sanders[47] appropriately notes, although research continues to clarify the important role of psychosocial risk factors in the development of disabling, chronic LBP, a number of significant issues need to be further resolved before such factors can be effectively employed in everyday clinical practice. As he states, "First, because the strength or weight of the predictability of a given risk factor is not really known, research into the comparative predictability of factors should be conducte Second, the aforementioned risk factors have yet to be clearly established as casual

TABLE 1.   Risk factors Associated with Chronic, Disabling Low Back Pain

- Elevation of MMPI scale 3 (hysteria)
- Depression
- Low activity / high pain behavior
- Negative beliefs / fear of pain
- Job dissatisfaction
- Blue collar / heavy physical work
- Older age
- Severe psychological stress or abuse
- High subjective pain intensity
- Substance abuse
- Receiving compensation and unemployment

From: Sanders SH: Risk factors for chronic, disabling low-back pain: An update for 2000. American Pain Society Bulletin 10:4-5, 2000.

in the development of chronic, disabling low-back pain. Third, it is essential to continue to explore the identification of addition risk factors" Obviously, additional research is needed to build upon the already firm foundation of factors that have been delineated.

REFERENCES

1. American Psychiatric Association: Diagnostic and Statistical Manual of Mental Disorders. Washington, DC, American Psychiatric Association, 1994.
2. Anderrson GBJ, Pope MH, Frymoyer JW, Snook SH: Occupational low back pain: Assessment, treatment, and prevention. In Pope MH, Anderrson GBJ, Frymoyer JW, Chaffin DB (eds): Epidemiology and Cost. St. Louis, Mosby Year Book, 1991.
3. Averill PM, Novy DM, Nelson DV, Berry LA: Correlates of depression in chronic pain patients: A comprehensive evaluation. Pain 65:93-100, 1996.
4. Banks SM, Kerns RD: Explaining the high rates of depression in chronic pain: A diathesis-stress framework. Psychol Bull 119:95-110, 1996.
5. Barnes D, Gatchel RJ, Mayer TG, Barnett J: Changes in MMPI profile levels of chronic low back pain patients following successful treatment. Spinal Dis 3:353-5, 1990.
6. Benson RC, Hanson KH, Matarazzo JD: Atypical pelvic pain in women: Gynecologic-psychiatric considerations. Am J Obstet Gynecol 77:806-825, 1959.
7. Bigos SJ, Battie MC, Spengler DM, et al: A prospective study of work perceptions and psychosocial factors affecting the report of back injury. Spine 16:1-6, 1991.
8. Bigos SJ, Spengler DM, Martin NA, et al.: Back injuries in industry: A retrospective study. Spine 11:241-256, 1986.
9. Blazer DG, Kessler RC, McGonagle KA, Swartz MS: The prevalence and distribution of major depression in a national community sample: The national comorbidity survey. Am J Psychiatry 151:979-986, 1994.
10. Blumer D, Heilbronn M: Chronic pain as a variant of depressive disease: The pain-prone disorder. J Nerv Ment Dis 170:381-406, 1982.
11. Brown GK, Nicassio PM: Development of questionnaire for the assessment of active and passive coping strategies in chronic pain patients. Pain 31:53-64, 1987.
12. Butler RW, Damarin FL, Beaulieu C, et al: Assessing cognitive coping strategies for acute postsurgical. Pain:139-153, 1989.
13. Cats-Baril WL, Frymoyer JW: Identifying patients at risk of becoming disabled because of low-back pain. Ther Vermont rehabilitation engineering center predictive model. Spine 16:605-607, 1991.
14. Croft PR, Papageorgiou AC, Ferry S, et al: Psychological distress and low back pain. Evidence from a prospective study in the general population. Spine 20:2731-2737, 1996.
15. Deyo RA, Cherkin D, Conrad D, Volinn E: Cost, controversy, crisis: Low back pain and the health of the public. Ann Rev Publ Health 12:141-156, 1991.
16. Dworkin RH, Handlin DS, Richlin DM, et al: Unraveling the effects of compensation, litigation, and employment on treatment response in chronic pain. Pain 23:46-59, 1986.
17. Engel GL: "Psychogenic" pain and the pain-prone patient. Am J Med:899-918, 1959.
18. Epker J, Gatchel RJ: Coping profile differences in the biopsychosocial functioning of TMD patients. Psychosom Med 62:69-79, 2000.

19. Fishbain DA: Secondary gain concept: Definition problems and its abuse in medical practice. Am Pain Soc J 3:264-273, 1994.

20. Fishbain DA, Goldberg M, Meagher BR, et al: Male and female chronic pain patients categorized by DSM-III psychiatric diagnostic criteria. Pain 26:181-197, 1986.

21. Flor H, Turk DC: Etiological theories and treatments for chronic back pain: I. Somatic models and interventions. Pain 19:105-121, 1984.

22. Fordyce W: Behavioral Methods of Control of Chronic Pain and Illness. St. Louis, Mosby, 1976.

23. Fordyce WE: Pain and suffering: A reappraisal. Am Psychol 43:276-283, 1988.

24. Gatchel RJ: Early development of physical and mental deconditioning in painful spinal disorders. In Mayer TG, Mooney V, Gatchel RJ (eds): Contemporary Conservative Care for Painful Spinal Disorders. Philadelphia, Lea & Febiger, 1991.

25. Gatchel RJ, Epker JT: Psychosocial predictors of chronic pain and response to treatment. In Gatchel RJ, Turk DC (eds): Psychosocial Factors in Pain: Critical Perspectives. New York, Guilford Publications, Inc., 1999, pp 412-434.

26. Gatchel RJ, Polatin PB, Mayer TG: The dominant role of psychosocial risk factors in the development of chronic low back pain disability. Spine 20:2702-2709, 1995.

27. Gatchel RJ, Polatin PB, Mayer TG, Garcy PD: Psychopathology and the rehabilitation of patients with chronic low back pain disability. Arch Phys Med Rehabil 75:666-70, 1994.

28. Gatchel RJ, Turk DC: Psychological Approaches to Pain Management: A Practitioner's Handbook. New York, Guilford Publications, Inc., 1996, .

29. Haley WE, Turner JA, Romano JM: Depression in chronic pain patients: Relation to pain, activity, and sex differences. Pain 23:337-343, 1985.

30. Haythornwaite JA, Sieber WJ, Kerns RD: Depression and the chronic pain experience. Pain 46:177-184, 1991.

31. Hodgkins AD, Watson JP: Psychiatric morbidity and illness in women with chronic pelvic pain. J Psychosom Res 38:3-9, 1994.

32. Holbrook T, Grazier K, Kelsey J, Stauffer R: The Frequency of Occurrence Impact and Cost of Selected Musculoskeletal Conditions in the United States. Rosemont, American Academy of Orthopedic Surgeons, 1984.

33. Jacobsen PB, Butler RW: Relation of cognitive coping and catastrophizing to acute pain and analgesic use following breast cancer surgery. J Behav Med 19:17-23, 1996.

34. Katon W, Egan K, Miller D: Chronic pain: Lifetime psychiatric diagnoses and family history. Am J Psychiatry 142:1156-1160, 1985.

35. Kerns R, Turk D, Rudy T: The West Haven-Yale Multidimensional Pain Inventory. Pain 23:345-356, 1985.

36. Kinney RK, Gatchel RJ, Polatin PB, et al: Prevalence of psychopathology in acute and chronic low back pain patients. J Occup Rehabil 1993:95-103, 1993.

37. Lanes TC, Gauron EF, Spratt KF, et al: Long-term follow-up of patients with chronic back pain treated in a multidisciplinary rehabilitation program. Spine 18:1103-1112, 1995.

38. Magni G, Moreschi C, Rigatti-Luchini S, Mersky H: Prospective study on the relationship between depressive symptoms and chronic musculoskeletal pain. Pain 56:289-298, 1994.

39. Mai FM, Merskey H: Briquet's treatise on hysteria: Synopsis and commentary. Arch Gen Psychiatry 37:1401-1405, 1980.

40. Main CJ, Waddell G: A comparison of cognitive measures in low back pain: Statistical structure and clinical validity at initial assessment. Pain 56:287-298, 1991.

41. Mayer TG, Gatchel RJ: Functional Restoration for Spinal Disorders: The Sports Medicine Approach. Philadelphia, Lea & Febiger, 1988.

42. McMahon MJ, Gatchel RJ, Polatin PB, Mayer TG: Early childhood abuse in chronic spinal disorder patients. A major barrier to treatment success. Spine 22:2408-15, 1997.

43. Melzack R, Wall PD: Pain mechanisms: A new theory. Science 50:971-979, 1965.

44. Polatin PB, Kinney RK, Gatchel RJ, et al: Psychiatric illness and chronic low-back pain. The mind and the spine—Which goes first? Spine 18:66-71, 1993.

45. Polatin PB, Kinney RK, Gatchel RJ, Lillo E, Mayer TG: Psychiatric illness and chronic low-back pain. The mind and the spine--which goes first? Spine 18:66-71, 1993.

46. Romano JM, Turner JA: Chronic pain and depression: Does the evidence support a relationship? Psychol Bull 97:18-34, 1985.

47. Sanders SH: Risk factors for chronic, disabling low-back pain: An update for 2000. American Pain Society Bulletin 10:4-5, 2000.

48. Schofferman J, Anderson D, Hines F, et al: Childhood psychological trauma correlates with unsuccessful lumbar spine surgery. Spine 17:S138-S144, 1992.

49. Schofferman J, Anderson D, Hines R, et al: Childhood psychological trauma and chronic refractory low-back pain. Clin J Pain 9:260-265, 1993.

50. Sternbach RA: Pain patients: Traits and treatment. New York, NY, Academic Press, 1974.
51. Sternbach RA, Wolf SR, Murphy RW, Akeson WH: Traits of pain patients: The low-back "loser."
    Psychosomatics 14:226-229, 1973.
52. Sullivan MJ, Stanish W, Waite H, et al: Catastophizing, pain, and disability in patients with soft-
    tissue injury. Pain 77:253-260, 1998.
53. Tait RC, Chibnall JT, Richardson WD: Litigation and employment status: Effects on patients with
    chronic pain. Pain 43:37-48, 1990.
54. Turk D, Rudy T: Toward an empirically derived taxonomy of chronic pain patients: Integration of
    psychological assessment data. J Consult Clin Psychol 56:233-238, 1988.
55. Turk DC Okifuji A: Directions in prescriptive chronic pain management based on diagnostic charac-
    teristics of the patient. American Pain Society Bulletin 8(5):5-11, 1997.
56. Turk DC, Rudy TE: Towards a comprehensive assessment of chronic pain patients. Behav Res Ther
    25:237-249, 1987.
57. Vingard E, Alfredsson L, Hagberg M, et al.: To what extent do current and past physical and psycho-
    logical occupational factors explain care-seeking for low back pain in a working population? Spine
    25:493-500, 2000.
58. VonKorff M, Simon G: The relationship between pain and depression. Br J Psychiatry Suppl 30:101-
    108, 1996.
59. Weickgenant AL, Slater MA, Patterson TL, et al: Coping activities in chronic low back pain: Rela-
    tionship to pain and disability. Pain 53:95-103, 1993.
60. Weisberg JN, Vittengle JR, Clark LA, et al: Personality and pain: Summary and future directions. In
    Gatchel RJ, Weisberg JN (eds): Personality Characteristics of Patients with Pain. Washington, D.C.,
    American Psychological Association, 2000.
61. Williams RA, Pruitt SD, Doctor JN, et al.: The contribution of job satisfaction to the transition from
    acute to chronic low back pain. Arch Phys Medi Rehabil 79:366-374, 1998.

DAVID C. RANDOLPH, MD

USE OF FUNCTIONAL EMPLOYMENT TESTING TO FACILITATE SAFE JOB PLACEMENT

From Private Practice
   Occupational Medicine and
   Disability Determination
   Millford, Ohio

Reprint requests to:
David C. Randolph, MD
   5724 Signal Hill Center
   Milford, OH 45150

Functional testing has undergone a significant evolution over the past several decades. It originally was designed to monitor individuals after significant trauma or substantial medical afflictions such as stroke.[1, 12, 19, 29, 30] Functional testing consisted primarily of observing individuals performing a variety of activities of daily living or attempting to lift objects of varying sizes of weights. Over the course of time, substantial changes in the mechanics of functional testing have occurred. In the present state of the art, functional testing is virtually a separate industry, with a high variation in types of functional testing and equipment available to perform these tasks.[29] The variation in this equipment ranges from the simplistic and technologically unadvanced, to extremely expensive instrumentation with protocols consisting of sometimes secretive and formulaic computerized devices.[29]

Presently, functional testing has a variety of uses in the employment arena, including safe job placement, post-injury evaluation, and appropriate screening for progress through various therapies. It is also used in various wellness programs.[12] With the advent of the American with Disabilities Act (ADA) in 1990, as well as other legislative issues (including equal employment opportunity and civil rights), the use of functional testing has taken on new vitality in the occupational setting. The functional capacity evaluation (FCE) now stands in some jurisdictions as a mainstay of safe job placement and risk diminution by (theoretically) providing objective data pertaining to an individual's ability to safely perform job tasks. Certainly it takes into consideration motivational issues and effort, when properly performed.[29]

It is clear from the direction legislative issues have taken over the past 10 years that there is a critical need for objective testing of an individual's functional abilities prior to assigning him or her to a workplace or permitting a return to previous job activities. The FCE also is useful in this capacity, to qualify and quantify the impact of pre-existing medical problems and conditions, as well as evaluate the impact of injurious events from a variety of causes. Controversy about functional testing presently centers on several issues: the need for a variety of differing types of functional testing, depending upon the unique employment setting; the confusion regarding the wide variation and types of functional testing available; the considerable lack of clarity with respect to the types of testing available; and the generalized confusion surrounding mechanics and interpretations of these evaluations.[29]

This chapter helps clarify some of these issues and provides the practitioner with[1] a guide to the current status of functional tests,[2] information on how the tests may best be used to monitor any individual through the pre-employment, post-injury recovery phase, and[3] tips for returning the worker to safe, sustained, remunerative employment.

THE ADA AND OTHER LEGISLATIVE ISSUES

The ADA prohibits employers from discriminating against qualified individuals with a disability, who are nonetheless capable of performing a job despite their health problems, with or without accommodations.[12] Industry in general expected and anticipated this legislation to have a major impact on its ability to function. Fortunately, the impact (while substantial from the standpoint of altering methods for assessing employment, employability, medical screening, and health evaluation) has been limited and largely centered around employment-related issues only.

The ADA includes a number of provisions which impact the screening of individuals with respect to prospective employment. Here are two:

- Prior to making a job offer, medical examinations and inquiries are not permitted except to the extent that the prospective employer may present to the prospect a description of the job tasks and query the individual as to their opinion pertaining to their ability to safely perform these tasks. A prospective employer may, under these circumstances, demonstrate the job site/tasks to the prospective employee and even have the employee perform such tasks to assure their abilities to perform these tasks in a safe fashion.
- An employer may make a conditional job offer and test the person before he or she actually begins work activities.

Several problems exist with this scenario. It is conceivable that in an attempt to make a good impression, the prospective employee will overexert and produce an injury while attempting to perform a task for which he or she is not suitable. The performance of such staged activities over a brief period of time does not confirm the prospective employer's capability of aerobically functioning to that capacity for an 8-hour day, 5 days a week. Finally, if the prospective employee is attempting return-to-work activities after an injury, staged job activity may not adequately and accurately represent that individual's safe work capacity.

From a post-offer perspective, the employer may receive information that conflicts with the individual's presumed functional capabilities. The employer cannot rescind the job offer unless it can be demonstrated that performance of such job duties poses a significant health threat to the prospective employee or other workers (direct threat).

Queries pertaining to additional medical history are limited pre-exam and must be job related, except for voluntary health programs (wellness programs) or those examinations mandated by Federal Law (e.g., Department of Transportation physicals, respirator physicals).

The concept of pre-placement or pre-employment testing has created confusion. The National Institute of Occupational Safety & Health (NIOSH) has provided five separate criteria for evaluating employment screening programs. These criteria include:

1. Is the test safe to administer?

A key issue in establishing safety during functional testing is avoidance of overexertion in the overly motivated or deconditioned candidate. This could occur in the candidate who is motivated by financial or personal concerns to return to some level of work for which he or she may not be adequately prepared, physically or emotionally.

2. Reliability

This term relates to the extent to which the results can be reproduced. Reproducibility is vital in all circumstances, because if a test is performed on one day and then repeated two or three weeks later, the change in the results needs to be definitively aligned with a change in the person's physical status, not with a change in the examiner or the equipment used. This is especially true in complex tasks such as manual dexterity and isokinetic testing.

3. Content Validity

A test is valid if the measured function can be equated to the job being evaluated. Specifically, if the goal is to test back strength, grip strength testing has no place. The content validity of any specific functional test must be demonstrated through job analysis. Therefore, an objective evaluation of the job tasks is mandatory, and the testing must adequately address those tasks. Otherwise, the testing will have no "content validity" and will be "invalid" with respect to evaluating an individual's ability to perform a certain task. If cut-off scores or standards are applied, these must be statistically validated with the use of normative data that is scientifically obtained for that work force.

4. Practicality

This addresses the need for minimizing expense with respect to the job tasks to be tested. Issues of practicality include evaluation of the total cost of the test being performed, the hardware required, and the personnel cost for administration.

5. Utility

Does the functional test relate to actual job performance? The utility criterion addresses whether the test is predictive, or is well correlated with actual job requirements. While some of these factors are epidemiologic in nature and may be burdensome and expensive in their performance, this can often become the most difficult criteria to achieve. Consider pre-employment back x-rays, often used in the past. They are costly, have limited predictive value, and expose the prospective employee to unnecessary radiation.

It is axiomatic that fitting a square peg into a round hole is not only difficult, but damages either the peg or the hole. Similarly, placing an individual into a job for which he or she may not be physically qualified increases the risk to the employer and the employee of costly injuries.

The Federal standards and guidelines herein described allow the employer and the employee to achieve a "proper fit." That is, if the employee understands the job requirements, the employer accurately and adequately presents the job demands, and a functional evaluation of the employee indicates a "match," then there is a substantial likelihood that injuries will be minimized and production capabilities substantially increased. There is some data available in the scientific literature to verify that this is in fact the case. Individuals who have been screened carefully demonstrated diminished frequency and intensity of injuries and lost time. Both employer and employee benefit when there is cautious evaluation and job placement using a proven scientific method.

FAULTY FUNCTIONAL TESTING

Functional testing generally has focused on screening individuals after various traumatic or medical events (e.g., motor vehicle accidents or strokes). Such "testing" has been highly variable, from a simple handshake testing grip strength to observations of activities of daily living. Rejection, with respect to the performance of certain tasks, has often been based on limited information obtained from a health screen questionnaire or a cursory physical exam. Too often, individuals have been accepted or rejected based on insufficient, nonobjective information. Treating health care personnel (including medical physicians, chiropractors, physical therapists, company nurses, and occupational therapists) have been asked with greater frequency to complete functional residual capacity forms indicating the physical capabilities of an individual who is attempting to return to work or to enter a new work arena. Often, the reported functional capabilities are based on subjective reports of the individual worker or a cursory physical examination consisting of range-of-motion studies or neurologic testing. This form of "data gathering" does not consider aerobic capacity, isokinetic or isometric strength capabilities, lifting capabilities, dexterity, agility, etc. Such modalities of functional assessment are suitable only for sedentary jobs or certain forms of work requiring only light physical demands. They are certainly far from sufficient when evaluating individuals for greater physical demand activities in the workplace.[3,4,5,6,9,11,13,15]

Unfortunately, this all too common practice has resulted in mere "guesstimates." An employment candidate may be asked what weight he or she can comfortably lift or carry, and an estimate of this weight is forthcoming based on the estimated weight of a bag of potatoes or a gallon of milk. While such a procedure may be helpful when work activities are not physically demanding, it is woefully insufficient when the worker is to be an "employed athlete," with physical demands of a highly aerobic nature, oftentimes requiring awkward postures and prolonged, demanding tasks. These activities may push the worker to the extremes of physical comfort.[13,22,24,28]

Such "guesstimates" are not only unscientific, but unreasonable, and serve to impede the normal employment process or return-to-work/transitional process. Problems arise for a variety of reasons: **1)** If the person's physical capabilities are overestimated by the health provider, then his or her ability to return to work may result in recurrent injury because of expectation of physical activity for which they have not been prepared. The recovery process may therefore be delayed. **2)** If the individual's work activities are underestimated, then there may be no work to which that individual may return. For example, if an individual works in a foundry, and the health care provider indicates he is capable of lifting only 10 pounds 8 weeks after a soft tissue back strain, such limited work activities may be unavailable, and the individual may be maintained in a "disabled" status for an unnecessarily prolonged length of time. Either scenario places the health care provider, employer, and employee in an untenable situation, with all parties on the losing end. Grabbing functional capabilities "out of thin air" without the benefit of scientific testing poses an unfair scenario which could very easily result in recurrent injury, delayed recovery, or anger directed toward the health care provider.[27,28]

The use of a valid and reliable functional test can alleviate this scenario. There are a variety of functional tests that are available to ease this set of sometimes uncomfortable circumstances; provide reproducible data for all parties involved; and promote more rapid and safe job placement and return to work after injuries.[29,30] The following is a brief discussion of one area of functional testing.

Example: Evaluation of Material Handling Capabilities

The *Dictionary of Occupational Titles*[18] references lifting capabilities as the key physical demand factor in the classification of work demands. This emphasis has produced a variety of "physical demand characteristic levels" which are now considered industry standards:

- Sedentary work: Lifting no more than 10 pounds as a maximum. Mostly sitting, but some standing or walking. Lifting may include articles such as dockets, ledgers, and small tools.
- Light work: Lifting a maximum of 20 pounds, with a frequent lift of up to 10 pounds. Mostly sitting, but standing and walking occur more often.
- Medium work: Lifting a 50-pound maximum, with a frequent lift of up to 25 pounds.
- Heavy work: Lifting up to 100 pounds maximum, with a frequent lift of up to 50 pounds.
- Very heavy: Lifting in excess of 100 pounds and/or frequent lifting of objects weighing up to 50 pounds or more.

It is important in evaluating lifting capabilities that individuals be tested at a variety of different lifting levels, including lifting from floor to knuckle to shoulder height, or shoulder to overhead. The amount of lifting to be performed varies, depending on the physical demand required for a particular job. In the performance of the lifting tasks, it is mandated that the individual being tested be closely observed by a skilled and experienced health care provider, who ensures that the tasks are done in a safe fashion, with good body mechanics and avoidance of dangerous postures. Advancement of lifting to higher levels should only be permitted when such lifting can be performed in a safe fashion, and the tested individual does not demonstrate unsafe behaviors and has not exceeded his or her functional capabilities.

If the test is terminated mid-session, the reasons should be documented. Reasons may include:

1. The evaluator discontinued the test because the evaluee had poor coordination or demonstrated poor body mechanics and had difficulty achieving a lift in a safe fashion at the level noted.
2. The evaluee voluntarily terminated the tasks as he or she did not wish to risk injury (the load was too heavy).
3. The test was terminated because the evaluee reached the stated maximum for the job being tested (for example, the tested maximum for a particular task was 40 pounds and the individual achieved that, or the evaluee reached or exceeded the parameters set by the treating physician).
4. The evaluee reached or exceeded the NIOSH-recommended load for the task designed.

Functional testing may also address aerobic capacity for physiologically demanding jobs. An adequate and properly performed job analysis will provide a statement pertaining to the MET demand for the particular task. The evaluee is tested following accepted protocols to determine aerobic capability and the ability to perform job tasks at that MET level. Continuous 8-hour exposure to job tasks should not exceed 33% of the individual's aerobic capacity as tested (*NIOSH Work Practice Guide for Manual Lifting*).

Aerobic capacity can be tested in a variety of fashions. The most common method is treadmill testing with monitoring of pulse and blood pressure. Maximum aerobic capacity testing is the most valid mechanism for determining aerobic capacity. However, maximum testing is usually not practical in the workplace. Maximum testing also mandates physician supervision to avoid the risk for coronary insult or additional injury (e.g., to the knees).[21–28] Consequently, submaximal testing, performed on a stair step or a treadmill, often is employed. A bicycle ergometer also can be used to determine aerobic capabilities.[29] Treadmill and step testing are similar from a physiologic standpoint to walking and lifting, and provide information that is easily translatable to workplace activities. Consequently, this information may be more valuable than that obtained from a bicycle ergometer.

COMPONENTS OF FUNCTIONAL TESTING

Tolerance for other activities is also mandatory if an individual's capabilities of performing job-associated tasks are to be completely tested. These activities include standing, walking, sitting, bending, twisting, stooping, crouching, crawling, reaching, and hand manipulation. Use of a variety of differing testing devices may be warranted, depending on circumstances. Such devices may include some standard tests, such as the Minnesota Rate of Manipulation or Purdue Pegboard

Clearly, functional testing must require some evaluation of the individual's basic physical characteristics. In addition to vital signs, height and weight become important, especially in narrowed assembly areas. An individual who must work in a seated posture without the ability to change position must have the physical characteristics to adjust to this. A 350-pound individual may not be able to suitably perform work activities under those circumstances, or sit in the same type of chair that a coworker weighing 150 pounds can use.

It is equally vital to evaluate an individual's functional range of motion with respect to involved or appropriate body parts—especially in the rehabilitative arena (for example, with injured workers who have had rotator cuff surgery or repair of torn knee ligaments). Document active range of motion. Girth measurements should accompany this to identify neuromuscular status and/or atrophy, or even to use as a baseline or follow-up measure in post-injury cases. Note that range of motion must be performed according to standards provided by the American Medical Association's *Guides to the Evaluation of Permanent Impairment*. Although this is not the only document outlining the correct performance of range of motion studies, it is certainly the most widely used.[2]

TYPES OF FUNCTIONAL TESTING

All functional capacity evaluations are not equal, and all do not provide the same types of information. In general terms, functional testing may be performed for a variety of differing reasons, including functional goal setting, disability rating, job task matching, occupational matching, and work capacity evaluation.[29] Occasionally an "a la carte method" is necessary when an individual need does not fit into any single category.

Functional goal setting is performed to set recovery goals and measure consequences of existing impairment. This type of functional testing includes evaluation of strength and range of motion. In general terms, it is used to provide an index of the performance to gauge clinical progress.

Disability rating measures loss of performance in key functional areas of work. This type of evaluation may be used to assess disability, as opposed to impairment, from a functional standpoint.

Job task matching evaluates the adequacy of a worker's ability to perform the essential functions of a given task. A formal job analysis should accompany this to determine specific physical demand requirements. Any functional impairment is determined from a physical exam. The information from this type of functional test is individualized.

Occupational matching matches the functional capability of a worker to various occupational demands. Such occupational demands are derived from the *Dictionary of Occupational Titles*.[18] The functional capacity evaluation becomes more complex because such occupational classifications contain all job tasks within that classification. The performance target then becomes the maximum for all tasks within a given job classification.

Work capacity evaluation is the most comprehensive and time consuming. There is no clear occupational target. The focus is very broad and may involve simulated work activities. Often such an evaluation exceeds a full 8-hour day.

INTEGRATION

The functional capacity evaluation can provide a plethora of information pertaining to the individual's physical capabilities. It is attendant on the health care provider to use this information to provide adequate job placement and help quantify the rehabilitative progress.

Functional testing can demonstrate an individual's level of safe physical performance and better direct the potential employee to a task for which he or she is suited. For example, an individual who demonstrates poor body mechanics when attempting to lift 40-pound objects overhead would be found during functional testing to be unsuitable for that task and would therefore not be recommended for such a task. If a prospective employee performs a certain job task during pre-placement testing safely and without difficulty, then he or she clearly qualifies for the performance of that task. If the potential employee's abilities are questionable or substandard, then the health care professional is in an excellent position to make an assessment pertaining to that individual's capabilities of performing that task, even to the extent of accompanying that person to the perspective job site and observing the performance of that task. If the individual is not a safe candidate for that task, then other recommendations can be made.

The impact of such a program is obvious. The employee benefits by avoiding an injury. The employer benefits by avoiding extensive costs related to injuries, as well as secondary loss of production. The result is a classic "win-win" situation.

Another pragmatic approach to the functional test involves assessing impairment and disability in individuals who have reported injuries of differing types. Such injured workers may present to an evaluating physician with limited functional capabilities of unclear etiology. These injured workers may be self-limited because of fear of recurrent injury, or may be symptom magnifying or malingering. Observations by a skilled examiner during the course of a functional evaluation can help sort out these issues.

The self-limiting injured worker demonstrates cooperation, but diminished function with altered body mechanics based on fear of injury. The diminished function is noted to be limited to the injured body part only. Magnifying or malingering workers often demonstrate a completely different clinical picture, with inconsistent performance and suggestions of manipulative behavior designed to demonstrate disability for secondary gain. Again, emotional issues representing underlying psychological conditions also can be observed by the examiner in a functional test.[6]

Functional testing can be repeated throughout treatment to determine progress through treatment and determine when the individual has reached maximum medical improvement. This data then can be compiled to determine if the individual is capable of returning to the previous level of employment, or should be referred for alternative employment.[29] This objective evaluation may be presented to the injured worker and used to help demonstrate to them in an objective fashion their clinical progress. It also can be used to limit unnecessary treatment and demonstrate to the injured worker that his or her status has remained at a point where it can no longer be predicted to improve.

CONCLUSION

Evaluation of functional capabilities has undergone a considerable evolution over the past several years. Despite the rapid growth in functional testing over the past few years it remains a young science with parameters which still need definition. Nevertheless, properly performed functional testing by skilled individuals, with cautiously selected test protocols appropriate for the particular needs of the employer and employee, can result in better and safer job placement and fewer injurious events, as well as more rapid return to safe workplace activities.

REFERENCES

1. Harvey RF, Jellinek HM. Functional performance assessment: A programmed approach. Arch Phys Med Rehab 1981; 62:456–461.
2. Luch JV, Jr., Florence DW. A brief history and comparative analysis of disability systems and impairment rating guides. Orthop Clin North Am 1988;19:839–844.
3. Mayer TG, Gatchel RJ, Keeley J, Mayer H. Optimal spinal strength normalization factors among male railroad workers. Spine 1993;18(2):239–244.
4. Mayer TG, Tenser AF, Christopherson S, Mooney V. Quantification of lumbar function, Part I. Spine 1985;10(8).
5. Mayer TG, Tenser AF, Christopherson S, Mooney V. Use of non-invasive techniques for quantification of low back dysfunction patients. Spine 1984;9(6).
6. Waddell G. Main CJ. Assessment of severity in low back disorders. Spine 1984;9(6).
7. American Medical Association. Guides to the evaluation of permanent impairment, 4th ed. AMA, 1993.
8. Wickstrom RJ, Evaluating physical qualifications of workers and jobs. In Bhattachara A, McGlothin JD (eds): Occupational Ergonomics. New York, Marcel Dekker, 1996.
9. Sacks BL, Ahmad SS, LaCroix M, et al: Objective assessment for exercise treatment on the B-200 Isostation as part of work tolerance rehabiliation. Spine 19(1)49–52.
10. Clark WL, Holdeman S, Johnson P, et al: Back impairment and disability determination. Spine 1988;13(3)332–341.
11. Dusic LA, Menard MR, Cooke C, et al: Concurrent validity of the ERGOS work simulator versus conventional functional capacity evaluation techniques in a workers' compensation population. J Occup Med 1993;35(8).
12. Matheson, LN. In Demeter SL, et al (eds): Disability Evaluation. St. Louis, Mosby, 1996.
13. Keeley J, Mayer TG, Cox R, et al: Quantification of lumbar function, Part V. Spine 1986;11(1).
14. Kohles S, Barnes D, Gatchel RJ, Mayer TG. Improved physical performance outcomes after functional restoration treatment in patients with chronic low back pain. Spine 1996;15(12):1321–1327.
15. Mennard MR, Cook C, Lock SR, et al: Pattern of performance in workers with low back pain during a comprehensive motor performance evaluation. Spine 1994;19(12):1359–1366.
16. Mostardi RA, Noe DA, Kovacik MW, Porterfield JA: Isokinetic lifting strength and occupational injury. Spine 1992; 17(2):189–193.
17. Newton M, Wadell G. Trunk strength testing with isomachines. Spine 1993;18(7):801–811.
18. U.S. Department of Labor Employment and Training Adminstration. Dictionary of Occupational Title, 4th ed. Washington, DC, US Government Printing Office, 1977.
19. Velozo CA. Work evaluations: Critique of the state of the art of functional assessment of work. Am J Occup Ther 1993;47:209–230.

20. Waddell G, McCulloch JA, Kummel E, Venner RM. Non-organic physical signs in low back pain. Spine 1980;5(2):117–125.
21. Wheeler DL, Graves JE, Miller GJ, et al: Functional assessment for prediction of lifting capacity. Spine 1994;19(9):1021–6.
22. Gross MT, Dailey ES, Dalton MD, et al: Relationship between lifting capacity and anthropometric measures. J Orthop Sports Phys Ther 2000; 30(5):237-47; discussion 258–61.
23. Jay MA, Lamb JM, Watson RL, et al: Sensitivity and specificity of the indicators of sincere effort of the EPIC lift capacity test on a previously injured population. Spine 2000; 25(11):1405–12.
24. Marras WS, Granata KP. Changes in trunk dynamics and spine loading during repeated trunk exerations. Spine 1997; 22(21):2564–70.
25. Moreland J, Finch E, Stratford P, Balsor B, Gill C. Interrater reliability of six tests of trunk muscle function and endurance. J Orthop Sports Phys Ther 1997; 26(4):200–8.
26. Lagerstrom C, Nordgren B. On the reliability and usefulness of methods for grip strength measurement. Scand J Rehabil Med. 1998; 30(2)113–9.
27. Kaplan GM, Wurtele SK, Gillis D. Maximal effort during functional capacity evaluations: An examination of psychological factors. Arch Phys Med Rehabil 1996; 77.
28. Sanders RL, Beissner KL, McManis BG. Estimates of weight that subjects can lift frequently in functional capacity evaluations. Phys Ther 1997; 77(12):1717–28.
29. King PM, Tuckwell N, Barrett TE. A critical review of functional capacity evaluations. Phys Ther 1998; 78(8):852–66.
30. Wyman DO. Evaluating patients for return to work. Am Fam Physician 1999; 59(4):844–8.

INDEX

Entries in **boldface type** indicate complete chapters.

Statement of Ownership, Management and Circulation
(Required by Section 3685, Title 39, United States Code)

1. Title of publication: OCCUPATIONAL MEDICINE: State of the Art Reviews
2. Publication number: 0885-114X
3. Date of filing: September 11, 2000
4. Frequency of issue: Quarterly
5. Number of issues published annually: 4
6. Annual subscription price: $99.00
7. Complete mailing address of known office of publication: Hanley & Belfus, Inc., 210 South 13th Street, Philadelphia, PA 19107
8. Complete mailing address of headquarters of general business office of publisher: Hanley & Belfus, Inc., 210 South 13th Street, Philadelphia, PA 19107
9. Full names and complete mailing addresses of publisher and managing editor: Publisher: Jacqueline Mahon, Hanley & Belfus, Inc., 210 South 13th Street, Philadelphia, PA 19107
    Managing editor: Jacqueline Mahon, Hanley & Belfus, Inc., 210 South 13th Street, Philadelphia, PA 19107
10. Owner: Hanley & Belfus, Inc., 210 S. 13th St., Philadelphia, PA 19107
    Holtzbrinck Publishing Holdings Limited Partnership, 415 Madison Ave., New York, NY 10017
11. Known bondholders, mortgagees, and other security holders owning or holding 1 percent or more of total amount of bonds, mortgages or other securities: None
12. Special rates: N.A.
13. Publication name: OCCUPATIONAL MEDICINE: State of the Art Reviews
14. Issue date for circulation data below: July–September 2000
15. Extent and nature of circulation:

	Average no. of copies ea. issue during preceding 12 months	Actual no. copies of single issue published nearest to filing date
A. Total no. copies (net press run)	2000	2000
B. Paid circulation:		
1. Sales through dealers, carriers, street vendors, and counter sales	–	–
2. Mail subscription	1090	1090
C. Total paid and/or requested circulation	1090	1090
D. Free distribution by mail	6	6
E. Free distribution outside the mail	36	36
F. Total free distribution	42	42
G. Total distribution	1132	1132
H. Copies not distributed		
1. Office use, leftovers, spoiled	868	868
2. Return from news agents	–	–
I. Total	2000	2000
Percent paid and/or requested circulation	96.28	96.28

I certify that all information furnished on this form is true and complete.

Linda C. Belfus, President